"Proving that fitness is more than skin deep, *BASIC Steps to Godly Fitness* points you to the whole person including your relationship with God. Laurette's 21-day Step-UP Program puts results at your fingertips. The combination of a worshipful attitude and physical activity turn the mundane into marvelous."

Marita Littauer

President, CLASServices
speaker and author of
But Lord, I Was Happy Shallow
and *Your Spiritual Personality*

"Finally! Fitness for spirit, soul and body made easy! In *BASIC Steps* Laurette combines solid biblical principles with the latest science to help you get and *stay* in shape. Humorous, encouraging, insightful. A book on a serious topic with a light touch. Delightfully doable!"

Florence Littauer

Founder, The CLASS Seminar
speaker and author of *Personality Plus* and *Silver Boxes*

"*BASIC Steps to Godly Fitness* is BASIC training for every person who desires balanced lifelong whole person wellness. Humorous and thought-provoking, Laurette gives us a straightforward look into her own life struggles, fears, disappointments, and ultimate victory for achieving Godly Fitness. Her use of God's Word as our source of authority, providing the foundation and principles for living wisely, and as a framework for understanding God's rules and life application, is masterfully and relevantly done. Truly a Whole Person Wellness guide. Own it...live well by it!"

Jim Nash

Founder/CEO of Healthy Initiative Ministries
(Christian Wellness Association & WellLIFE Centers)

"My first experience with Laurette's PraiseMoves program was while looking for a Christian alternative to yoga on the Internet. I read Laurette's testimony and ordered her entire program. I have been experiencing terrific results using PraiseMoves personally and have been recommending it to all of my patients ever since. I am thankful to Laurette for designing a program that combines Christ-centered worship with the physical benefits often attributed to yoga. Now, *BASIC Steps to Godly Fitness* will be a wonderful addition for me to promote to my patients as a well-rounded approach to spiritual and physical health. Insightful, informative, and in touch!"

Steven J. Scafidi, D.C.

America's Chiropractic Center, New Jersey

"Laurette Willis wrote *BASIC Steps to Godly Fitness* for people like me who just want the basics. Her advice is practical and flexible without being restrictive. Nurtured by the Scriptures, her humor and encouraging words keep you on track. The three-week Step-UP Program offers daily doses of action—one BASIC step at a time!"

Karen Robertson

speaker and author of *Raising Kids Right*

"I am pleased to recommend *BASIC Steps to Godly Fitness.* This book is the kind of resource we recommend to our members looking for a Christ-centered approach to optimal health. Laurette's honesty and openness are refreshing as she challenges us to 'renew our minds!' Her approach to prayer, praise, and fasting will encourage you. In a day when we appreciate that spiritual fitness is as important as nutrition and exercise for the health of the whole person, we need more resources like this one."

Rev. Ron Lively

Executive Director, Christian Wellness Association
Founder and Executive Director, Medical Mobilizers

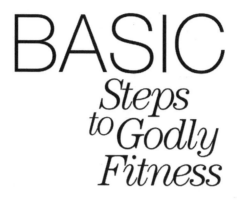

BASIC
Steps to Godly Fitness

Laurette Willis

HARVEST HOUSE PUBLISHERS

EUGENE, OREGON

Readers are advised to consult with their physician or other medical practitioner before implementing the suggestions that follow. This book is not intended to take the place of sound medical advice or to treat specific maladies. Neither the author nor the publisher assumes any liability for possible adverse consequences as a result of the information contained herein.

Cover by Koechel Peterson & Associates, Inc., Minneapolis, Minnesota

Cover photo © Ron Chapple/Thinkstock/Getty Images

BASIC STEPS TO GODLY FITNESS
Copyright © 2005 by Laurette Willis
Published by Harvest House Publishers
Eugene, Oregon 97402
www.harvesthousepublishers.com

Library of Congress Cataloging-in-Publication Data
Willis, Laurette, 1957-
   BASIC steps to godly fitness / Laurette Willis.
      p. cm.
   ISBN 0-7369-1565-6 (pbk.)
   1. Health—Religious aspects—Christianity.   I. Title.
   BT732.W55 2005
   248.4—dc22   2004024319

Printed in the United States of America

05 06 07 08 09 10 11 12 / VP-CF / 10 9 8 7 6 5 4 3 2 1

This book is dedicated to my precious parents, Charles and Jacqueline Cronin, who so eagerly demonstrated they loved their little girl with all their hearts. I am grateful for your love, delightful humor, keen intellects, and appreciation for the sweet things of life. I miss your laughter, but I know I will see you "over yonder."

I offer special thanks to my dear husband, Paul, for his patient heart, unwavering faith, and constant prayers. You are my warrior and my prince. I love you.

A sincere thank you goes to Christian authors and speakers Florence Littauer and Marita Littauer of CLASServices.com for their selfless giving, encouragement, and example.

Special thanks to those whose prayers light my way: Nola Jeanne Baird, Gene Ruth Brumbach, Pastor Donna Allen, Pastor Arlis and Elizabeth Moon, and many others who would hit me if I wrote their names in a book. You know who you are. I love you dearly.

Contents

Bad News,
Good News

I HATE THE WAY I LOOK!" "Why can't I get the weight off? I've tried *everything!*" "I feel like a prisoner trapped in this body." "Why can't I stop overeating? I have no control around food." "O God, help me!" Have you ever said or thought some of those things?

You're not alone. Close to 65 percent of the American population is considered overweight (that's 6 out of 10 people you meet!), and 30 percent of Americans are considered obese (30 or more pounds over their ideal weight).[1]

According to the National Institutes of Health, overweight and obesity are known risk factors for diabetes, heart disease, stroke, hypertension, gallbladder disease, osteoarthritis, sleep apnea, breathing problems, and some forms of cancer (uterine, breast, colorectal, kidney, and gallbladder). Obesity is also associated with high blood cholesterol, complications of pregnancy, menstrual irregularities, psychological disorders (such as depression), and increased surgical risk.

Such alarming indicators of the state of our national health have had a devastating impact on health care.

The Wellness Council of America has stated that health care costs are at their highest point ever—and could reach $2 *trillion* by 2007! Many Americans have seven or more chronic ailments, and while we're the wealthiest nation spending more money on health care than any other, we are certainly not the healthiest.[2] Annual health care costs have gone from $141 per person in 1960 to approximately $4000 in 2004.

You may be thinking, *Okay, Laurette. Enough with the bad news already! I know that being overweight can affect my health. What can I do about it? I need help—and fast!*

The good news is that the majority of illnesses linked to overweight and obesity are entirely preventable. Even more importantly, we serve an awesome God, who has specifically designed you to succeed in every area of life. The Lord reminds us that "His divine power has given to us all things that pertain to life and godliness, through the knowledge of Him who called us."[3] He's already *given* us these things, and we attain them through knowledge of Him. You could say this about success for the Christian: It's a given!

God's plan for you includes optimal health at your ideal weight, energy, joy, and confidence—free from the bondage of overeating and guilt. How can I be so sure of that? I know because that is what God has done for me and countless others who have sought the Scriptures for the answers to seemingly impossible situations. In Jeremiah 29:11 God said, "'For I know the thoughts that I think toward you,' says the LORD, 'thoughts of peace and not of evil, to give you a future and a hope.'"

Perhaps you're thinking, *Yeah, I know that—but I've tried everything.* I thought I had too—especially everything man-made. I didn't see a way out. Then I realized that Jesus Himself said that He *is* the way.[4] He also said, "With men this is impossible, but with God all things are possible."[5]

I'd like to share with you part of my own journey of recovery from compulsive overeating, alcoholism, smoking, self-hatred, and the deception of the New Age movement to health and victory by following the BASIC Steps I'll share with you in this book. Then together we'll embark on a journey of recovery together step-by-step. I believe that with each small step, you'll experience for yourself the Lord leading you to victory.

Introduction

"Mommy! Mommy! I can't stop eating!" The little girl ran into her parents' bedroom and knelt beside the bed.

On that bright, beautiful mid afternoon in suburban Long Island, Mommy was asleep in her darkened bedroom.

The girl was small, a little pudgy, with dimpled hands and knees. Her round "Campbell kids" face was framed with a brunette pixie cut. Tears pooled in her bright amber eyes and flowed down chubby little cheeks as she patted Mommy's face.

The little girl her mother called "Little Laurie So-Sweet" had been eating bread and butter, Easy-Bake Oven cake mix, cereal, and anything else she could find to comfort her while Mommy slept. I was that little girl. I was six years old, and food was my friend.

Looking back at that day, I wonder if my mother was suffering from depression—or had she been drinking? When I was six I realized something was very wrong with Mommy and Daddy. Behind closed doors, the beautiful home on Long Island held secrets, alcohol, yelling, and tears.

I had what our Irish-American family called a "healthy appetite." I was a card-carrying member of the Clean Plate Club, and I *always* had room for dessert.

"Where do you put it all?" my father would tease me.

"In Coco," I'd reply. Coco was the huge white toy dog I'd had since I was a baby. I really shouldn't have blamed Coco. He was already stuffed.

At Northside Elementary School, the boys discovered I'd cry when they called me "Fatso." It became their favorite taunt. I remember many days running home from school in tears. An only child, I was unaccustomed to the teasing children often do. I didn't understand why they were so mean to me.

"I know what they're really saying," I'd tell my mother. "They're saying I have a fat soul, huh, Mommy?" It was a silly thing to say. I knew it wasn't true. I was just trying to ease the tension for both of us.

Once alone in my room, I'd look in the mirror and scold myself: "You're fat! You're ugly! I hate you! I hate you!" Then came the tears. After the tears came the search for food. I'd watch television and eat until I was numb. The unending cycle continued for more than 30 years.

I attempted my first diet when I was 11 years old. I saved up the money from my lemonade stand and secretly went to the neighborhood drugstore to buy a box of *amazing* Ayds weight-loss candies.

"These are for your mother, right?" the pharmacist asked, peering over his spectacles.

"Uh…yes," I lied.

The directions said I should eat one Ayds candy with a glass of water in place of a meal or for a snack. I ate half the box at one sitting and hid the rest under my dresser. They were delicious. I gained three pounds.

I'm surprised that I didn't become heavier than I did. I attribute this to my mother becoming the town's first "health-food nut," as people interested in nutrition were called in the 1960s. While other children's lunch boxes had Twinkies and Yodels with their bologna sandwiches on white bread, I had celery sticks and apple slices with my tuna sandwich on whole grain bread. I didn't seem to mind the kids' taunts about the weird food. I made it a game. I could eat carrot sticks like a rabbit and do an impression of Bugs Bunny to make them laugh. An audience! I loved it.

I noticed that when Mom was following a healthy diet, taking vitamins, and exercising daily, she didn't drink alcohol as much—sometimes not at all, which was marvelous to me. She was fun to be around, and we loved being together. We'd giggle like girlfriends as we took long walks through the neighborhood holding hands. Acting out all the characters to the *Peter Pan* album I got for Christmas, we'd fly around the playroom singing "I Won't Grow Up." Snuggling together on the couch, we read *Little Women* aloud with English accents...

When I was seven years old my mother started practicing yoga. A nice-looking Asian couple had a popular daytime yoga program on television. It was scheduled right after Jack La Lanne's exercise show. It seemed so harmless, so relaxing, and so *spiritual.* Not familiar with the Bible or a Christian lifestyle (although we regularly attended church), neither Mom nor I understood the deceptive nature of yoga.

The exercises relaxed Mom. Since we did almost everything together, we did yoga exercises together too. When she began teaching free yoga classes to high school and college students in our home, I was the little demonstration model. I loved the attention. My father thought it was all rather kooky, but he was busy building his law practice and didn't pay much attention to what we did when he wasn't home.

For several years Mom and I visited an ashram (yoga retreat) in upstate New York associated with Swami Satchidananda. When I was ten years old, the swami visited the ashram while we were there and "blessed" me. He smelled sickeningly sweet. His long, wavy black hair was heavy with oil and always looked wet as it flowed over his saffron shoulders. Perhaps I was supposed to feel blessed by the attention. I just felt uncomfortable.

During meditation times, I wouldn't keep my eyes closed. I kept peeking at all the serene-looking adults in the room as we sat cross-legged in the lotus posture, incense filling the air. I liked doing the exercises better.

After becoming a Christian in 1987, I looked back at our seemingly innocent introduction to yoga as the open door that gave the enemy entrance into our lives. From the ages of 7 to 29 I was involved in the New Age movement. I tried everything from yoga to channeling spirits, from reading crystals to psychism, from tarot cards to pendulums. I even gave readings at psychic fairs occasionally—keeping a Bible on the table for looks! Oh, what a merciful God we serve! I studied various religions, tasting them like a smorgasbord: Hinduism, Buddhism, Zoroastrianism, "mystic" Christianity, Kabala, Taoism, Sufism, Unity, Universal Mind, and Unitarianism.

I've since learned, however, that the only way to God is through faith in Jesus. God's way is perfect, and His plan for you is perfect. By following God's ways in the Bible, you can experience a peace that nothing else can give you. The apostle Paul reminds us, "When I am weak, then I am strong."[1] In fact, when I take even the smallest of steps in the right direction and ask God to help me, He rushes up to meet me. He will make up the difference between what you can do and what He can do. And that is good news!

Take a step. That's the key: Choose to take one simple step, and then *do* it.

God has set before you "life and death, blessings and curses. Now choose life.... For the LORD is your life."[2]

Before we take our first step together toward higher fitness, let's take a quick look at what fitness is and what it is not.

Fitness for His Witness

"If the LORD delights in a man's way, he makes his steps firm; though he stumble, he will not fall, for the LORD upholds him with his hand."[3]

Fitness for the Christian is more than physical health. Dictionaries define fitness as the state of being physically sound and healthy, but I have found that godly fitness also brings freedom. If we consider freedom to be the ability to do God's will without any hindrances, fitness takes on a whole new meaning. I call it "Fitness for His Witness" and offer seminars by the same name at churches and women's conferences throughout the country. During these seminars, participants discover that fitness is more than skin deep.

Why is fitness godly? I believe, with the apostle Paul, "You were bought at a price; therefore glorify God in your body and in your spirit, which are God's."[4] By learning to take good care of the wonderful bodies He's given us, we can honor Him. I like to think godly fitness reflects our desire to glorify Him by pursuing spiritual, emotional, and physical fitness.

BASIC (Body And Soul In Christ) Scriptural Foundations

You are comprised of three parts: body, soul, and spirit. Likewise, godly fitness includes three BASIC parts. Body And Soul In Christ.

You are a spirit, you have a soul, and you live in a body.

Let's look at the scriptural evidence. Paul made the division clear when he prayed for the church in Thessalonica, "May your whole spirit and soul and body be kept blameless until that day when our Lord Jesus Christ comes again."[5]

First, you are a spirit: "Since Christ lives within you, even though our body will die because of sin, your spirit is alive because you have been made right with God."[6]

Second, you have a soul: "For the word of God is living and powerful, and sharper than any two-edged sword, piercing even to the division of soul and spirit."[7]

Third, you live in a body: "Or don't you know that your body is the temple of the Holy Spirit, who lives in you and was given to you by God? You do not belong to yourself, for God bought you with a high price. So you must honor God with your body."[8]

Perhaps most importantly, as Christians, we are in Christ as perfectly as He is in us. "In Him we live and move and have our being."[9]

If you have not asked Jesus Christ to come into your heart and give you a new life, or if you haven't been enjoying a heart-to-heart relationship with the Lord who made you, I invite you to turn to page 221. If you are unsure whether or not that means you, it does. I'll be right here waiting for you when you get back.

What You Will Learn in *BASIC Steps to Godly Fitness*

For your body: You will discover simple steps to incorporate better nutrition and fitness into your daily life to bring results that last—and improve your family's health as well.

For your soul: You will learn how to overcome destructive thought patterns, make healthy choices, and discover the freeing power of forgiveness (an important key to answered prayer).

For your spirit (in Christ): You will see how you can grow in your relationship with God. Prayer, praise, and fasting will set you on the fast track to a lifetime of victory—not only in areas of weight loss and fitness but also in family relationships, healing from past hurts, and fulfilling your purpose in God's plan for you.

I'm as excited as you are to experience the wonderful things the Lord has in store for us as He leads us step-by-step on this journey of recovery and total restoration in Him. God is so good!

Step One

✧⋅✦

Body And Soul In Christ

1

Eating What's Right *Will Solve What's* Wrong

*E*ATING WHAT'S RIGHT? *But I thought diets were all about what* not *to eat."* I hear you. Having been a compulsive overeater since childhood, I rebelled against the "don'ts" of dieting. I may have succeeded at following a diet for a few days, but I looked for loopholes and opportunities to sneak around the rules. If the rules said, "Don't eat that," I countered with, "Oh yeah? Just watch me!"

I'm sure you were never that bad, but did you ever think while on a diet, *I've been so good, I deserve a little reward?* Sound familiar? For some of us the little reward turned into an episode of "Lost Weekend in Bingeville." I figured that since I already ate half the carton of ice cream I might as well polish the rest of it off. *What's the use? I'm hopeless,* I thought. Burying the empty container in the trash, I'd dash out to the store to replace it before anyone noticed I'd eaten the whole thing. I could fool the family, but my waistline told another story.

Over the years, well-meaning persons offered suggestions about my choice of food. One might suggest, "How about eating a salad instead?" I'd grit my teeth and think, *How about minding your own business?* A less timid soul might have voiced their replies aloud, but all I could do was think them. I'll never forget one relative's remark at an outdoor birthday party when I was 12 years old. As I reached for a slice of cake, she said, "Honey, you don't want to get fatter, do you?

Why don't you have a nice piece of celery instead?" I was so astonished (and hurt) by her words that I grabbed the slice of cake and ran to the garden shed to hide and eat the cake through my tears.

I was unable to offer a snappy comeback at the time, but I would go over and over these encounters in my mind, dazzling my offenders with clever retorts and cutting remarks.

Just like the alcoholic who "drinks at" the person who has angered him or the situation that troubles her, the compulsive overeater "eats at" her adversary or troubles, numbing herself with food to stuff down the hurt and anger. I discovered overeating was a convenient distraction, a form of procrastination. As long as I was stuffing myself with food, I didn't have to face the real problem—at least not now. I'll start the new diet on Monday, or after the holidays, or when things slow down, or when the kids go back to school, or—you fill in the blank.

In *BASIC Steps*, we're not going on another diet. We're not getting on another program or crusade or wagon we can just as easily fall off. Instead, we're going to sow some seeds—healthy choices that help build our character—from which we will reap a harvest of positive changes physically and emotionally. We'll also be sowing seeds to develop the fruit of the Spirit in our lives, knowing that "whatever a man sows [or plants], that he will also reap."[1]

Focus on What You *Can* Do

We experience great freedom when we focus on what we *can* do instead of what we should not do. When Jesus was asked by a scribe which was the greatest commandment of all, Jesus answered by giving two powerful, positive directives that cover all the bases: "Love the Lord your God with all your heart, with all your soul, with all your mind, and with all your strength.... Love your neighbor as yourself."[2] In other words, if you're doing the right things—loving God first and foremost and loving others with a pure heart—you will be keeping all of the commandments.

If you have children, you've seen this principle at work. Tell me which statement elicits a better response from a child: "You cannot go to the movies, and that's final!" or "Which two friends would you like to invite over to play this afternoon?"

A Step in the Right Direction

If you will purpose to do four simple things every day, you will be taking some important BASIC Steps in the areas of health and nutrition. Some days you may achieve all four, some only one—or none—but remember, you're not jumping on and off a diet. There's no wagon to fall off. You're sowing, watering, and nurturing seeds of health, faithfulness, and patience for a future harvest. You may notice positive changes immediately, or you may not.

I believe the first triumph you will experience is simply knowing you are taking a step in the right direction. You will have a calm assurance that says you are making progress. And *progress,* not perfection, is the key.

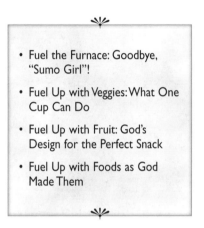

- Fuel the Furnace: Goodbye, "Sumo Girl"!

- Fuel Up with Veggies: What One Cup Can Do

- Fuel Up with Fruit: God's Design for the Perfect Snack

- Fuel Up with Foods as God Made Them

Fuel the Furnace: Goodbye, "Sumo Girl"!

We have a woodstove in our home and enjoy the warmth it radiates on a cold winter night. However, I have yet to see it give off any heat without us first adding the fuel it needs—wood. The same is true with our bodies. We can't expect our bodies to burn fat unless we eat. "But I've *been* eating—that's my problem," I often hear. But the problem is not the act of eating itself. You need to eat. God designed your body that way. It has more to do with *what* and *when* you are eating.

Part of the answer to why skipping meals doesn't help us lose weight can be learned from Japanese sumo wrestlers.

Quick Quiz #1:
How do sumo wrestlers get so big?

Japanese sumo wrestlers may be the world's top experts in how to gain weight. They are devoted to gaining as much weight as possible because the heavier the wrestler, the more likely he is to beat his opponent.

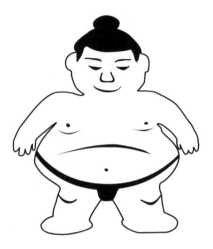

If you want to lose weight, you'd be wise to learn from the sumo wrestler what *not* to do. Here is how an average 165-pound man becomes a formidable 400-pound contender. His day looks something like this:

He lives in a dormitory-style sumo training center with other athletes like himself and awakens around 6:00 A.M. For the next four or five hours he trains and exercises without eating.

Clue: Skipping breakfast will not *make you slender.*

Most overweight people do not eat breakfast. I was one of them—until I realized I was becoming a sumo girl. Skipping breakfast makes one more likely to overeat later in the day. It also causes a 5 percent drop in metabolism. No wonder I was so sleepy!

A sumo wrestler exercises a lot, so you'd think he'd lose weight. But his eating habits ensure that he keeps piling weight on regardless of how heavily he trains for competition.

Clue: Exercise alone will not cause you to lose weight. You must change your eating habits.

The sumo wrestler's first meal of the day is around noon, after which he takes a nap for three or four hours. His trainers want him to conserve as much energy as possible so that most of the calories he eats will be stored as fat.

Clue: Going to sleep after eating puts on weight. In order to lose weight, do not eat within three hours of bedtime.

To gain the large belly for which sumo wrestlers are famous, he eats only two meals a day.

Clue: Infrequent meals equal weight gain. Eat smaller amounts every three to four hours instead.

Some women have told me, "I shouldn't be so heavy. I only eat twice a day." So do sumo wrestlers. You'd think they were nonstop eating machines to become so huge. But no, they eat just two meals a day—two *huge* meals a day. The average sumo meal would feed five or more average eaters!

Clue: Portion sizes do count.

In order to train his stomach to eat those huge portions, he eats past the point where he is no longer hungry. He continually ignores his "full signal."

Clue: If you want to lose weight, stop eating when you are no longer hungry—rather than when you feel full.

The sumo wrestler's diet is surprisingly healthy and low in fat. He eats the same dish at every meal: *chanko-nabe,* a meat stew with rice and vegetables. This traditional sumo dish is eaten with very little variation every day, twice a day.

Clue: Don't be a boring eater.

I used to call myself a boring eater until I decided to stop calling myself names. We get into a rut with our eating sometimes, don't we?

Fitness experts agree we should vary our workouts because the muscles adapt quickly. If we continue to exercise the same exact way all the time, the body becomes accustomed to it and we won't experience the progress we'd like. Similarly, we should add variety to our food plans. This isn't just to fend off boredom at the dinner table. When you eat a variety of different foods, you are more likely to get the broad range of nutrients your body needs. You also won't get that horribly deprived feeling of being on a diet and become tempted to go running into the arms of the nearest Keebler Cookies elf.

To avoid becoming a sumo girl, remember this:

- Skipping breakfast will not make you slender. You must eat breakfast.

- Exercise alone will not cause you to lose weight. Eating habits must change.

- Going to sleep after eating puts on weight. Do not eat within three hours of bedtime.

- Infrequent meals equal weight gain. Eat smaller amounts every three to four hours.
- Portion sizes do count. Use a measuring cup until you can estimate accurately.
- Stop eating when you are no longer hungry, not when you're full.
- Don't be a boring eater. Variety is the spice of life!

Fuel Up with Veggies: What One Cup Can Do

Five to nine servings of fruit and vegetables every day will nourish our bodies, help prevent disease, and control our weight. That means another helping of French fries and tomato ketchup for most Americans, but not for those of us seeking godly fitness!

The USDA estimates Americans are eating 20 percent more vegetables now than 35 years ago *(hooray!)*, but the increase is mostly in potatoes—half of that amount in French fries *(boo!)*. The close of the twentieth century saw the largest consumption of French fries ever— roughly 28 pounds of fries per person per year! Considering that some of us seldom eat French fries, some folks are eating more than their share (perhaps two or three times as much). No wonder the obesity rate has climbed so dramatically over the years.

What is one serving of raw vegetables? It's one cup of raw leafy vegetables, or a half a cup of chopped raw vegetables. A serving size is generally what you can fit into your hand.

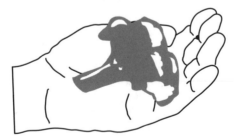

If you are not eating any raw vegetables at all, start with one cup. If you are already eating a cup or two, add another cup (it's really a lot less than you might think).

A great way to get a couple of servings of veggies into your family's diet is to have one or two cups of a simply prepared salad at each person's dinner place setting. But don't go for the cellophane-wrapped iceberg lettuce. According to the March 2004 *Journal of the American Dietetic Association,* the most popular fruits and vegetables (corn, potatoes, iceberg lettuce, apples, and bananas) are not necessarily the most nutritious. Typically, the darker the color of the vegetable, the higher the nutrient content will be.

Go for Color!

Green: Leafy greens (spinach, lettuces, collard, mustard and turnip greens), asparagus, green peppers, broccoli, green beans, peas, green cabbage, Brussels sprouts, okra (not fried!), zucchini, green onions, cilantro, parsley, cucumber, celery, sprouts

Yellow and orange: carrots, corn, pumpkin, yellow peppers, sweet potato, butternut squash, summer squash, spaghetti squash (our favorite!)

Red: tomatoes, red cabbage, red peppers, red onions, beets

White: cauliflower, onions, garlic, mushrooms, parsnips, shallots, turnips

Blue and purple: eggplant

Cruciferous vegetables such as broccoli, cauliflower, cabbage, Brussels sprouts, bok choy, and kale contain many nutrients, including glucosinolates (don't worry, there won't be a test on this!), which are being shown to lower cancer risk. (For those who enjoy the origin of words as much as I do, *cruciferous* means "cross bearer." It comes from the Latin word for *cross* and refers to these plants' leaves or petals, which form the shape of a cross.)

According to the American Institute for Cancer Research, laboratory studies have demonstrated that eating cruciferous vegetables helps control an intricate system of bodily enzymes that protect us against cancer. What's even more exciting is that elements of these "cross-bearing" vegetables have been shown to *stop the growth* of cancer cells, including tumors of the breast, endometrium, lung, colon, liver, and cervix. This is good to know because the American Cancer Society's 2005 annual report reveals that cancer has surpassed heart disease as the leading cause of death in the United States.

In our home we rarely have a salad without raw broccoli and cauliflower. For my salad dressing I use organic apple cider vinegar (a natural antibiotic that aids digestion and weight control) and flaxseed or walnut oil (rich in essential fatty acids). My husband prefers Italian dressing, so I add a teaspoon of flaxseed oil to his salad with the dressing he likes.

In a perfect world we'd stroll out the back door, pluck a juicy orange or peach off a tree, and gather organic vegetables and herbs from our garden for a tasty salad. But for most of us, it's off to the supermarket for our family's food needs.

Organically grown produce (without pesticides or chemical fertilizers) has become the choice for many shoppers. Even though a higher price tag comes with the USDA certified organic seal, most dyed-in-the-wool shoppers of organic foods believe the price is worth it to ensure their families are not ingesting toxic pesticides in their food. Whether you decide to go organic or not, be sure to wash all produce thoroughly.

Be willing to try new things. Never tried a raw spinach and veggie salad? Think you might hate it? We all have certain prejudices against food we *think* we don't like (and ones we really do dislike, of course). I remember a childish prejudice I had against zucchini (Italian squash). I tried to feed my portion to our Shetland sheepdog, Lady, but she wouldn't eat it either. While zucchini still won't make me do backflips in the produce aisle, I've learned that lightly steamed zucchini and other veggies with cheese and herbs tastes great (and it's good for me too!).

Dare to Sprout Your Own!

No matter where you live, you can grow crunchy, delicious sprouts in three to five days. Sprouts are loaded with disease-fighting phytochemicals, antioxidants, and antiaging compounds. Sprouts are great in salads, sandwiches, or stir-fry meals. All you need is a sprouting jar (or make your own with a jar, cheesecloth or piece of hosiery, and a rubber band to cover the jar opening), and some sprouting seeds from your health food store. Good sprouting seeds are alfalfa, mung beans, Chinese cabbage, and radish.

Soak the seeds for six to eight hours in your sprouting jar. Keep them in a dark place—but not so out of sight that you forget about them! I put mine in one of the cupboards I open frequently. Under a dish towel on the kitchen counter is also a good place.

After soaking, rinse the seeds in the jar, drain them well, and then set the jar on its side. I also put it in a bowl to elevate the base of the jar. Excess moisture drains out the sprouting jar lid. Make sure the seeds are not all clumped up in one space. Spread them out a bit to aerate them. Rinse them two to three times a day. On the third or fourth day expose them to indirect sunlight for three to five hours so the chlorophyll in the sprouts will turn them green. Now they're ready to eat.

Sprouts can be placed in a sealed plastic bag or jar and refrigerated for several days. Some people like to rinse them once a day to help sprouts maintain their crispness, but mine don't seem to stay in the refrigerator more than a day or two. We eat 'em up!

I was a former city dweller who had never planted more than pumpkin seeds in a cup for a fifth grade science project, so my first sprouting experience was semi-monumental. "It works!" I yelled to my husband, Paul. Obviously charmed by my exuberance, Paul quipped, "You'll be beaming with vitality in no time!"

Comfort or Style? Nutrition or Lollipops?

Have you noticed the desire for comfort replaces the fascination with style as you get older? In the early '80s I had a pair of silver shoes with platform heels six and a half inches tall—*dancing* shoes! All my girlfriends were taller than I was, so to keep from being called Shorty, I wore those ridiculous pumps when we went out to the discos (this was my B.C. lifestyle!). But now, give me a pair of lace-up tennis shoes, and I don't care *what* you call me.

Perhaps good nutrition will become more important than how good something tastes as we mature too (lest we live on lollipops and ice cream sodas, and leave earth before our time). The amazing thing is that the "cleaner" you eat (eating more foods as God created them, fewer processed foods, and saner portions), the more your taste buds prefer the healthier fare.

Another vegetable on my grown-up hit parade has become spaghetti squash. Even Paul, the Pasta Prince of our household, loves it. As the name implies, it looks a lot like spaghetti when cooked, and it is so simple to make. Treat it just as you would cooked spaghetti, and even the kids will be willing to set aside macaroni and cheese once in a while for this healthier alternative. See the recipe section for my *easy* BASIC Steps SpaghettiOs! recipe.

Fuel Up with Fruit: God's Design for the Perfect Snack

Are you already eating one piece of fruit? Make it two. Add some variety. When was the last time you made a big fresh fruit salad for the family? Check out the fruit smoothies and kid-tested Ice Dreams in the recipe section.

If you *really* want some spring in your step, eat one piece of fruit alone or added to a BASIC Power Shake (in the recipes section) in the morning and then have a piece of fresh fruit as a mid-morning or mid-afternoon snack. By eating two pieces of fresh fruit and a big raw veggie salad with lunch or dinner, four or five servings of the recommended five to nine will be raw, uncooked produce.

Many low-carb dieters will turn up their noses at the suggestion of fruit for a snack when they can have a highly processed snack bar with artificial flavors and colors, unpronounceable ingredients, and questionable nutritive value—but with only five net carbs and a three-year shelf life! Hmmm. What's wrong with this picture? I fell for the same line. Looking at the snack bar's fine print, however, revealed 220 calories (90 calories from fat). I'd bought into the big sign on the label that said "Three Grams of Net Carbs" as if it meant the bar had only three *calories!*

One medium apple may have 17 net carbohydrate grams, but it's packed with vitamins, minerals, fiber, and all the natural *zing* God

---

Who Says Ketchup and Fries Aren't Found in Nature?

A neighbor of mine noticed his potato plant had begun sprouting *tomatoes!* Ed had been growing vegetables for years but had never seen anything like this before. His potato plants grew potatoes underground and tomatoes on the vines above the ground.

A state horticultural expert told him the two plants are related, and the birds may have cross-pollinated them, causing the confusion. Who knows, potato-tomatoes could become a whole new fast-food sensation.

Why do I want to sing, "Hold the pickle, hold the lettuce..."?

put in there from the get-go. It has only 81 calories, no fat, and no assembly required. It's notable, tote-able, and even quotable ("An apple a day…")! Okay, okay, I know—I shouldn't play with my food.

Good for You

Why is eating fresh fruits and vegetables so important? Well, when was the last time you read about an important disease-fighting component being found in a candy bar or French fries or a box of sugared cardboard (cereal)? Fruit and vegetables contain important immune-boosting phytochemicals and antioxidants.

Phytochemicals are plant chemicals that contain protective, disease-preventing compounds. They are not classified as nutrients because they're not necessary for sustaining life, but they're associated with the prevention and treatment of at least four of the leading causes of death in the United States—cancer, diabetes, cardiovascular disease, and hypertension.[3]

Phytochemicals help prevent both cell damage and cancer cell reproduction, and they decrease cholesterol levels. Researchers have discovered more than 900 different phytochemicals, and they continue to discover more. Believe it or not, there may be as many as 100 different phytochemicals in just one serving of vegetables![4] Now doesn't that sound like something God would make?

Antioxidants act as cell protectors against damaging cell by-products called free radicals, which we'll discuss in our section on avoiding processed foods. If left unchecked, free radicals weaken the immune system and may cause cancer, heart damage, diabetes, and premature aging.

Antioxidants do amazing work. They bind themselves to free radicals and transform them into harmless compounds (I wonder what would happen if you poured some on a rebellious teenager? Hmmm…).

Antioxidants repair damage done to cells. Not surprisingly, the highest concentrations of phytochemicals and antioxidants are found in the most deeply or brightly colored fruits and vegetables. Remember to go for color!

When should you eat your fruit snack? Why not take an apple or orange with you if you work outside the home? I find a juicy Fuji apple or crisp Red Delicious around 2:30 or 3:00 p.m. is great to ward off that 3:00 to 5:00 p.m. slump. Isn't that usually the time we hear the Three Musketeers or Keebler elves calling our name? Keeping some little snack-packs of mixed fruit or applesauce in your desk at work or cupboard at home can stave off the Cookie Monster; and though a mini-box of raisins has more concentrated fruit sugar than an apple, it's still better than a candy bar.

Convenience Foods vs. Making Healthy Food Convenient

If you make healthy choices convenient, you and your family are less likely to opt for poor quality, highly processed convenience foods when your blood sugar is low and you're not thinking as clearly. I learned a long time ago in a 12-step program for compulsive overeaters to follow the wisdom of "HALT." "HALT" meant we were to never allow ourselves to become too hungry, angry, lonely, or tired. When we experience any of these states, our reserves are low and we're apt to make poor choices. With food, that usually means going for whatever comes to a dull mind first, or whatever is close at hand. Having fruit nearby can keep us from a binge.

Fuel Up with Foods as God Made Them

As much as possible, eat foods in their natural state (as God made them), limiting processed foods.

Quick Quiz #2:
Which meal is closest to its natural state?

a. fresh fruit cup, raw vegetable salad with lemon juice (or apple cider vinegar and flaxseed oil), whole wheat tortillas with beans and steamed veggies

b. raw veggie salad with "lite" salad dressing, cooked salmon with lemon juice, frozen veggies with cheese, brown rice, fruit dessert

c. iceberg lettuce and tomato with sweet and creamy Italian dressing, instant macaroni and cheese (just add water!), canned peas, Sara-licious Put-On-the-Pounds cake

d. fast-food burger (with lettuce, tomato and pickle— those *are* vegetables, aren't they?), French fries (medium-size, I'm watching what I eat), frozen dessert (what *is* that anyway?), diet soda (to wash it down quickly please, I'm driving)

Did I read anyone's mail? I wrote from memory, believe me. You may have noticed our menu became increasingly more processed and further away from its natural state as our list progressed.

Okay, we're *modern* people; we don't live in ancient times. How can we possibly do what Jesus would do when it comes to food? Actually, it's a lot easier than you think. You know what has helped me make changes in this area? Knowledge. Before anyone said "knowledge is power," God said through the prophet Hosea, "My people are destroyed for lack of knowledge."[5] Both knowledge (information) and wisdom (understanding how to apply that knowledge) are valuable, necessary, and available.

Let's look at one of the blights of modern life: processed food. Some of you may be thinking, *But processed foods are convenient! I thought conveniences were blessings, not curses!* True—thanks to the joys of technology, most of us don't have to till the soil, grind the wheat, and kill the fatted calf to feed our family. I'll admit I'd rather reach for a box of raisins at the supermarket than grow, harvest, and dry the grapes myself. Many conveniences are blessings.

Certainly not all processed foods are bad for us either. In fact, processed food is mentioned in the Bible. Bread (processed grain) is mentioned as early as the third chapter of Genesis. Bread is meant to be a blessing; otherwise Jesus would not have referred to Himself as "the bread of life."[6]

But as food moves further from its original state, the more processes it goes through. More preservatives and chemicals are added to increase its shelf life, and it has less nutritional value for our bodies to use. Also, these nonfood items become potentially harmful as our bodies struggle under the weight of the toxic load.

Yeah, but It Costs More

According to the Economic Research Service of the USDA, Americans can meet the recommendation of three servings of fruits and four servings of vegetables daily for 64 cents per person. Sixty-four cents a day! That's only $2.56 for a family of four to receive 12 servings of fruit and 16 servings of vegetables. That's about half the cost for only one person's fast-food hamburger, fries, and cola. Seems like a better investment to me.

We're going to pay for health one way or the other. We can either *invest* time and money up front for fitness and nutrition, or we can *spend* time and money later trying to fix what's already been broken. I'm told good investments have good returns. Even if you're recovering from an illness, you have many months and years ahead to enjoy a healthy return on the investments you make today. You *can* make the rest of your life the best of your life.

Yikes! Beaming New-Age Energy Waves?

While I was still a New Ager before I became a Christian, I would often eat with fellow metaphysical folks like myself who would hold their hands over the greasy fast food and "pray" that the gunk in it would be neutralized by the energy flowing from their hands. How different is that from the Christian who "blesses" the Super-Dooper-Sized Belly Bomber and fries with the 64-ounce Acid Wash over ice? By the way, did you know you cannot "rebuke" a calorie or cast the fat out of a triple hot fudge sundae?

Would I be mistaken in suggesting some of us may be coming up hard against the third commandment by using the name of the Lord in vain over our food choices? I've been guilty of thoughtlessness in this area myself. I have looked at an unhealthy meal I was about to eat—knowing it was full of bad choices for me—and asked God to bless it "in the name of Jesus." At the same time, I'd sense that "check" in my spirit that something just wasn't right—and I knew it.

"My people are destroyed for lack of knowledge," we're told. How about the knowledge we recognize and choose to ignore? If you can't say amen, say ouch. I did.

The Results of Oxidative Stress

When we look at the word *antioxidant*, we know the prefix "anti" means "against." What then do antioxidants resist for us? Antioxidants resist the process of oxidation. Oxidation is what happens when an apple slice turns brown or metal rusts. Free radicals are unstable molecules that can damage stable molecules, leading to oxidation (oxidative stress).

We are exposed to free radicals when we absorb chemical additives or expose ourselves to sunlight. Even normal cellular processes produce free radicals. If we are not receiving sufficient antioxidant protection from fruits, vegetables, and dietary supplements, we can compromise our health.

Scientists have discovered that free radical damage weakens the immune system and is a leading cause of cancer, heart disease, and diabetes. And there's another cause for concern for those of us who don't want to look or feel older than we are. Oxidative stress may also be responsible for premature aging, wrinkling of the skin, stiffening of the joints, cataracts, and more.

Make the Exchange

When buying processed foods, go for foods with the least amount of chemicals and preservatives. I heard of a gal who won't buy anything with ingredients she can't pronounce. That sounds laughable, but it may not be such a bad idea!

Instead of soda pop, drink water (add lemon or a tablespoon of apple cider vinegar and a teaspoon of raw honey for taste, added nutrients, and enzymes)—or if you must have a carbonated beverage, try sparkling water. Make sure it's not sweetened with sugar or aspartame. Why? Here are some of the not-so-bubbly news items about sodas:

One can of regular soda pop has about ten teaspoons of sugar, 150 calories, 30 to 55 milligrams of caffeine, as well as artificial food colors and sulphites. But you say, "I drink *diet* soda." Some nutritional experts believe the artificial sweeteners are worse than sugar, and they may actually make you crave more sweets and fattening foods.

The findings of recent studies published in the *International Journal of Obesity* showed that eating and drinking artificially sweetened foods and beverages may be causing people to underestimate their caloric intake. Laboratory animals that ingested artificial sweeteners overate *three times more calories* than those that did not.[7]

Obesity rates in children seem linked to sodas as well. A study published in *The Lancet*, Britain's prestigious medical journal, states that for every soft drink or sugar-sweetened beverage a child drinks each day, his or her obesity risk jumps 60 percent.[8]

Water—a Miracle Elixir?

If you're looking for a miracle elixir, water may be the closest thing you'll find. The word *water* occurs 396 times in the Bible. It represents all that is clean, refreshing, wholesome, and life-giving. Notice that Jesus didn't say He would give believers the *iced tea* of life!

Please don't sell yourself short by saying, "I hate water." You may as well say, "I don't want to be healthy!" Even if you don't like water now, be patient with yourself. By following the BASIC Steps program, you can regain your God-given thirst for water.

Less Water Equals Fat Gain; More Water Equals Fat Loss

Water also seems to be the single most important catalyst in weight loss and maintaining a healthy weight. Decreasing water intake actually causes fat deposits to increase, while increasing water intake can reduce fat deposits. Why? The kidneys need water to function properly. When they are not receiving sufficient water, they're not operating at full capacity, and some of the load is managed by the liver. One of the liver's many functions is to metabolize stored fat into energy, but if it's doing some of the work of the kidneys, it's not able to function at maximum capacity. The result? The body stores more fat instead of metabolizing it.

Did you know that sometimes you only *think* you're hungry? You may actually be thirsty. I call it "mouth hunger." You know that sensation you have when you want something to eat but the desire isn't coming from your stomach? Perhaps you want to change a taste in your mouth, and you know that eating a particular snack will change it. Next time that happens, drink water instead (not soda pop, juice, coffee, or tea).

Many women have told me they are rarely thirsty. Our bodies can become imbalanced from eating food when we're really thirsty or drinking caffeinated soda, coffee, or tea, which further dehydrate the body. These physical imbalances can cause us to lose our natural thirst for water.

Water Retention Woes

What about water retention (edema)? Many women are concerned that drinking water will aggravate bloating and swollen ankles. Actually, the opposite is true. The best treatment for fluid retention is drinking sufficient quantities of water. Seems contrary, doesn't it? It's comparable to the "Fuel the Furnace" rule. When we don't eat sufficient quantities of food every few hours, the body perceives starvation, lowers metabolism to burn fewer calories, and hoards fat. Similarly, when the body isn't receiving enough water, it perceives this as a threat to survival. It holds on to as much water as it can and stores it in spaces outside the cells. This results in swollen feet, ankles, and hands.

Diuretics only worsen the condition. Stored water may be forced out for a time (along with nutrients the body needs), but the body will replace the water lost as soon as it can. Swelling returns, so diuretics are taken again and the cycle is perpetuated. If edema is a problem for you, first try decreasing salt and caffeine intake and increasing the amount of water you drink.

What Is a Sufficient Amount of Water?

"Does iced tea count?" "What about juice, coffee, or diet soda?" Even though juices and man-made beverages contain water, pure water is the only liquid that does not require the body to work to process it. Soft drinks have chemicals and colorings that have to be removed, and caffeinated beverages actually dehydrate the body, removing more water than the beverage contains.

Most nutrition experts agree that 64 ounces (eight eight-ounce glasses) of water each day is adequate for most people. If you're overweight, one eight-ounce glass is recommended for each additional 25 pounds of body weight.

Want an easier way to remember? Take your weight and divide it by two. Drink that number in *ounces* of water each day. For example if you weigh 160 pounds, half that number is 80. Drink 80 ounces of water every day (or ten eight-ounce glasses).

Unfortunately, our water supply is tainted by chemicals and waste matter even in the purest of settings. Today water must be filtered, so purchase a good water filtration system (preferably steam distilled) or buy bottled water. See www.BasicSteps.info for the system we recommend and use.

Don't like the taste of water? Filtration systems can do wonders, but until you can get one, refrigerating water improves the taste. Also try a squeeze of lemon, or two teaspoons of organic apple cider vinegar and a teaspoon of honey.

Increase the amount of water you drink when exercising, in warm weather, or if working outdoors. Cold water appears to be absorbed by the body more quickly and may even help burn more calories (we like that!).

If you stop drinking enough water, your natural thirst will disappear. Your body fluids will go out of balance, causing fluid retention and mysterious weight gain. The solution? Simply increase your water intake to 64 or more ounces per day.

For something so simple to be so beneficial, you know it must be created by God! Pure water and lots of it—it's God's miracle elixir!

A Delicate Subject

Some researchers estimate that 70 percent of the population experiences constipation. Drinking more water and adding fiber in the form of vegetables, fruit, and psyllium seed husks (one to two teaspoons daily) will increase regularity. This is vital because as you lose weight, excess fat and toxins leave the body as waste. If constipation is a concern, you will have a difficult time losing weight, and you may be developing more serious problems. Laxatives such as pills, herbal tablets, or teas do not help the situation in the long run. The body can become dependent on laxatives, causing normal bowel function to suffer. Healthy probiotic bacteria needed for proper intestinal function can be washed out of the system by continued laxative use, causing chronic constipation.

Ask at your local health food store for a good probiotic supplement such as acidophilus to replace the good bacteria in your system. One excellent probiotic supplement is Probiotic Restore made by AdvoCare. These probiotic organisms assist in waste removal, acting like little "scrubbies" on the inside of the intestines. They aid internal cleansing, digestion, and weight loss, and they help keep a good balance of healthy intestinal flora.

Antibiotics destroy the good bacteria with the bad, so if you've taken them, you need to take probiotics to maintain a healthy balance of good bacteria in your system.

While we're on the subject of intestinal health, did you know it's normal to have several bowel movements a day? I know that's not something we like talking about, but I have spoken with women who think one or two bowel movements a *week* is normal. It is not. Think of it—you eat several times a day, right? The excess food that's not used by the body has to go *somewhere*. If the body is not moving waste, it is being stored, often lining the walls of the large intestines. Since nutrition is absorbed all along the digestive tract, old waste coating the intestines can keep the body from absorbing nutrients. In addition to impeding weight loss, constipation can cause lethargy, headaches, acne, hemorrhoids, even cancer. If this is a concern, I urge you to speak with a qualified health professional.

God Made Low-Carb Bars—or Did He?

Net-carb mania! Boy, I sure fell for that one. Eating chocolate bars with "Only Three Net Carbs" on the wrapper became an addiction. It's as if the package read "Only Three *Calories*"! Something within us still jumps with hopeful anticipation at the claims of "Lose ten pounds in three days" or "No exercise, no dieting, no kidding...." And no difference either.

Regardless of what the bold little "Net Carb" circle says on the label, you should pay attention to the fine print in the Nutrition Facts section. Here's an example from a tasty chocolate syrup that boasts "*Zero* Sugar Carbs" and "0.6 Net Carbs per Serving."

Serving size . . . . 2 tbs

Calories per serving 120

Total carbs per serving. . . . . 26.4 grams

Net effective carbs per serving. . . . . 0.6 grams

How can something with 26.4 grams of carbohydrate end up with 0.6 grams net carbohydrates? The answer is found in claims that sugar alcohols such as maltitol and sorbitol produce a slower rise in blood sugar than regular table sugar. This is not a false statement, but it is misleading. Since they're still carbohydrates, the body will either use them as fuel or store them as fat. *Store them as fat?* They didn't tell us that on the label!

To get a more realistic look at what the low-carb treat will have on us, look at the total number of carbohydrate grams listed and divide by two. That will give you an idea of how many carbs are really going to affect your body, regardless of what the brightly colored circle says. In our chocolate sauce example, that would be around 13 grams. Any way you slice it, 120 calories in two tablespoons is still 120 calories in two tablespoons!

Remember that low-carb cookies, candy bars, and other treats are not meals. We're better off eating real, God-made food whenever possible.

A Fad by Any Other Name...

Over the years, our desire for the quick fix and "having our cake and eating it too" have spawned a deluge of diet books and fads, a gaggle of infomercials, and a plethora of profitable pills, potions, patches, and pudge-busters. Yet the obesity crisis in North America has continued to escalate.

When it comes to fad diets, I've decided FAD is an acronym for Fat-Adding Demon. Here's why. God designed muscle not only to give the body mobility and strength but also to burn fat. Muscle weighs more than fat, and muscle is often destroyed on fad diets. *Catabolism* results (sounds like *cannibalism*, doesn't it?). This is the process by which the body breaks down its own tissue for energy. Less muscle equals less fat burned. The body, perceiving starvation, is more interested in surviving than in making you look good in a bathing suit. The Lord designed your body so that when starvation seems imminent, your metabolism lowers and you burn less fat. This means you're more susceptible to gaining weight back quickly when you start eating normally again—and the weight gained back is fat, not muscle. Your metabolism can remain low for months after the crash diet is over, making your next diet more difficult because you have less muscle to burn calories. By continually jumping on and off diets, you can change your body composition drastically, gaining more fat and losing muscle—even if your weight does not increase sharply. This is where we get the term "yo-yo dieting." Sounds like a Fat-Adding Demon to me!

How to Spot a FAD (Fat-Adding Demon) Diet

Any diet that guarantees quick weight loss or overemphasizes one specific type of food has a good chance of being a Fat-Adding Demon diet. Avoid extravagant claims that promise you'll lose more than two pounds a week. These may seem to reduce weight quickly, but as mentioned previously, water and muscle are lost, and weight is regained as soon as the diet is over—often with extra pounds as well.

A prolonged FAD diet can cause more serious side effects, including dehydration, heart palpitations, and kidney problems.

Realizing that F-A-D is b-a-d, what really works? We've learned that *fast* doesn't *last*. That's why a quick fix is really a slow stall. It's just prolonging the pain until we decide to do things the right way—God's way. What *is* God's way? While God does work miracles, His way of teaching us what is right takes time—until we learn it.

I spent 30 years following a series of quick-fix diets to lose the same weight over and over and over again (and changing my body composition to less muscle and more flab each time I regained the weight). I was like the Israelites who wandered in the wilderness because they refused to enter the Promised Land. I knew what science, medicine, and the fitness experts had to say, but I wanted to avoid having to make sensible lifestyle changes. I wanted the "Abracadabra Diet"—poof! You're thin and can eat *anything* you want! I didn't want to use discipline, eat normal portions of food, say no to some foods, and exercise on a regular basis.

In addition to ignoring nutritional science and fitness rules, I ignored God's rules as well. What are His rules? "We do not want you to become lazy, but to imitate those who through *faith and patience* inherit what has been promised" (Hebrews 6:12 NIV, emphasis added).

People can harvest green fruit and vegetables and spray them with ethylene gas to force ripeness, but the ripening of the fruit of the Spirit cannot be forced. Maturity is a process. We take one step at a time, walking by faith and following the Lord. I've learned that anything that guarantees instant results offers empty promises. While FAD diets appear to work at first, good habits take time to develop. A healthful lifestyle isn't perfected overnight. It must be practiced over time.

That's why I wrote the Step-UP program in chapter 10 as an outline for healthy living rather than a rigid diet. You won't fail as long as you are taking a step forward. Remember, aim for progress, not perfection.

Lasting change comes as we grow in our relationship with the Lord, follow His promptings, and yield to the fruit of the Spirit within us. It does not come from a particular diet or exercise program. We succeed when we stop looking for a quick fix, give up

dieting, and start focusing on the Lord and His Word, cultivating the
fruit of faithfulness, patient endurance, and self-control. Your habits
will change—and so will you!

Bringing It Home

In this chapter, I learned this about…

fueling the furnace: _____

_____

fueling up with veggies: _____

_____

fueling up with fruit: _____

_____

fueling up with foods as God made them: _____

_____

I can start doing this better today: _____

_____

Lord, I ask You to help me _____

_____

2

Break*fast: It's a Command*

So when he had received food, he was strengthened.

ACTS 9:19

Have you ever thought about the word *breakfast* before? We're to break (or end) the fast (the abstinence from food) we've been on since our last meal the night before.

I like to see it as a command. Break your fast! Nutritionists and dieticians recommend eating your first meal of the day *no later* than one hour after awakening. "But I'm not hungry in the morning," countless women have told me. Part of the reason for that is eating late the night before and going to bed with undigested food on the stomach. I often woke up groggy and hungover after a late-night binge. The last thing I wanted to look at was food. Only around 10:00 A.M. would something like a donut or sugary muffin sound appealing. It starts a vicious circle. If you hate eating breakfast like I did, your blood chemistry may be out of balance first thing in the morning. Breakfast is just what your body needs to stabilize blood sugar and a queasy stomach.

One thing most overweight people have in common is that they seldom eat breakfast. (Remember the sumo wrestler's diet?) You start the day at a loss by not eating breakfast—a loss of energy, brain power, and memory as well as a 5 percent drop in metabolism. Not eating breakfast also provides a built-in trigger designed to cause overeating later in the day.

Proof That Breakfast Eaters Win—and *Lose!*

In 1992, Vanderbilt University conducted a survey with over-weight people who routinely skipped breakfast. When they began eating breakfast, they became big *losers*—losing an average of 17 pounds in 12 weeks. They were less hungry at other meals, and eating breakfast fired up their metabolism to burn more fat the rest of the day.[1]

As a struggling actor in New York City in the early 1980s, my eating habits left much to be desired. Late night snacking before I went to sleep caused me to wake up feeling exhausted instead of refreshed. Food? I couldn't think of it. Coffee—or a diet cola—was all I wanted before I was out the door to join thousands of other weary subway travelers on our way to work. A part-time secretarial job for an insurance company in the Wall Street area was how I supported "my acting habit," as I called it.

Often I wouldn't eat anything until lunchtime, surviving on a diet cola every few hours for that jolt of caffeine to keep me from falling face-first onto my desk. Sometimes there were muffins, donuts, or bagels around. I couldn't say no.

Eating lunch wasn't a huge priority, but I did like to get away from my desk. If I wanted to be "good" I'd eat a salad (loaded with high-calorie dressing). If I didn't care, I'd eat French fries, washing them down with more diet cola.

By 3:00 P.M. all I could think about was chocolate, cookies, and sugary frozen yogurt. By the time I left work at 5:00 P.M., I was a human steamroller. I mowed down anyone or anything that stood between me and my drug—food. *I've been so good today*, I reasoned with myself. *I hardly ate anything. I deserve it.* Like the gun sounding at the start of a sporting event, I had triggered my body to play the eating game. The problem was that I lost every time.

After several hours of snacking (or bingeing) in front of the television, sometimes having dinner and sometimes not, I'd go to bed. *I did it again*, I'd think, hating myself. *I'll start that diet tomorrow, or I just won't eat.* And the cycle continued.

After years of living with the consequences of unhealthy choices, I decided to change. The conversion has taken time, and I'm still in process. Now, by the grace of God, I can say that the healthier choice is most often my preferred choice. It *is* a choice. I wasn't forced beyond my control to improve my health—just as I hadn't been forced to ruin it. God leaves the choice up to us. I'd like to share with you some ideas that have helped me, trusting that the Holy Spirit will guide you in what will work best for you.

Bringing the Firstfruits of Your Day to the Lord

If you will devote the first 40 to 60 minutes of your day to the Lord in communion with Him, exercising and nourishing your spirit, soul, and body, you will be amazed at the transformation that will begin to take place in your life. The Step-UP program (chapter 10) can give you an outline.

The Lord told Moses that the children of Israel were to offer a portion of the firstfruits of their harvest as a sacrificial offering to the Lord.[2] Some people think that what happened in the Old Testament doesn't apply to our lives today. However, Paul said about the people of the Old Testament that "all these things happened to them as examples, and they were written for our admonition [or instruction]."[3]

As Christians, we realize that Jesus became the sacrifice for us.[4] We offer our bodies as *living* sacrifices,[5] and we offer sacrifices of praise to God or "the fruit of our lips."[6]

The sacrifices we offer to the Lord become holy. *Holy* means consecrated or set apart to God and separated from sin. The Bible tells us that "if the firstfruit is holy, the lump is also holy."[7] Paul was speaking of Israel, but can you see how offering the first part of your day to the Lord brings blessings all the rest of the day as well? Not sure? Try it. Tomorrow morning, spend the first part of your day in fellowship with the Lord. Exercise and nourish your spirit, soul, and body "as to the Lord,"[8] and see how smoothly the rest of the day will go for you. You will still have challenges, but you'll have the Lord's wisdom on what to do. By reading His Word and listening for His guidance first thing in the morning, you will be more sensitive to His leading all day long.

Breakfast Choices

In a perfect world, breakfast would be a leisurely time to enjoy a delicious, nutritious meal with the family and chat about everyone's plans for the day. Some families may be so blessed, but most of us are on the "Hurry up—I gotta get outta here *now!*" plan. A BASIC Power

Shake (in the recipe section) is an easy meal for those on the go. It's like a smoothie with muscle. Instead of a serving bowl of sugary breakfast cereal, which has little more nutrition than candied cardboard, make enough BASIC Power Shake for the whole family. Adding fruit such as a banana, frozen strawberries, or orange juice makes a healthy shake to suit each one's personal preference. If you'd rather not drink your breakfast, here are some more quick ideas.

- Include some simple carbohydrates (juice, fresh or dried fruit) for fast-start energy.
- Include some complex carbohydrates (cereal, bread, or whole grains) for sustained energy.
- Include some protein (eggs, meat, dairy, nuts, seeds, or soy) for muscle-building energy.

Examples

- ½ banana, ⅔ cup whole grain cereal, ½ cup skim milk
- Orange juice, slice whole grain toast, 2 scrambled eggs
- All-fruit jam, wheat muffin, 1 tablespoon almond butter or peanut butter

Get the idea? Now you try it. Think of what you have available in the kitchen right now. Write down two easy choices you could have for breakfast tomorrow morning that both you and the rest of the family would enjoy. See the recipe section for more breakfast ideas.

Note: If you have digestive problems (such as indigestion, gas, bloating, irritable bowel syndrome, or constipation), don't eat fruit with other foods. Try eating fruit first and then wait 20 minutes before eating the rest of your meal. Fruit digests quickly and will also help with elimination. Also, avoid eating starches (bread and potatoes) with protein (eggs and meat). God made us able to digest many types of foods, but if you are suffering from problems with digestion, the combinations of foods you are eating may be the culprit. If your body is not digesting food properly, you are probably not absorbing the nutrients from your food and dietary supplements as you should, which can affect your general health and energy as well.

If you suspect food allergies or sensitivities, do without wheat, coffee, tea, dairy, soy, corn, artificial sweeteners, and MSG from your diet for a month. Seek out a good nutritionist or dietician who can help you design a nutritious diet you and your family can enjoy.

Bringing It Home

In this chapter I learned…

1. _____

2. _____

3. _____

I can start doing this better today:_____

_____

Lord, I ask You to help me _____

_____

3

Success Strategies

Let food be your medicine and medicine be your food.

HIPPOCRATES

Success Strategy #1

From Food Pyramid to Food Circle: A New Paradigm

Let's get the most nutrition possible with the least number of calories. The more high-quality nutrition we take in with fewer calories, the more the body is getting what it needs to operate at maximum efficiency. Energy increases, so we're more active, and our body burns more fat. As energy increases, our attitude improves, and we're a lot more pleasant to be around. (You know how cranky you can be when you're tired!)

Which foods are high in nutrition and fiber and low in fat, calories, and chemical additives? Whole grains, fresh vegetables, fruit, and legumes form the core of the BASIC Steps food plan (with some nuts and seeds). Almost everyone is familiar with the USDA's Food Guide Pyramid, which is currently being redesigned to reflect the government's concern about the obesity epidemic.

One problem with the design of the Food Guide Pyramid is that our eye is naturally drawn to the top of the pyramid—the "use sparingly" fats, oils, and sweets section. The foundation is usually the last place we look (the grains group). We also have a tendency to think whatever is on top is best.

I suggest a new paradigm: The Food Circle. Our eye is drawn to the large center of the circle, where we find the nutrient-dense foods we are to eat in abundance. The rings become smaller as we move away from the center.

The nonfood items of our circle are equally important: Exercise and an Active Lifestyle, and Praise. These will be covered in later chapters. Interestingly, the USDA's January 2005 dietary guidelines now include exercise as an important part of a healthy lifestyle.

The Food Circle shows us that the majority of our nutrients are to come from whole grains, vegetables, fruits, legumes, nuts, and seeds. The model resembles the types of foods eaten in Mediterranean cultures where instances of heart disease, diet-related cancers, and obesity are far less prevalent than in the industrialized Western world.[1]

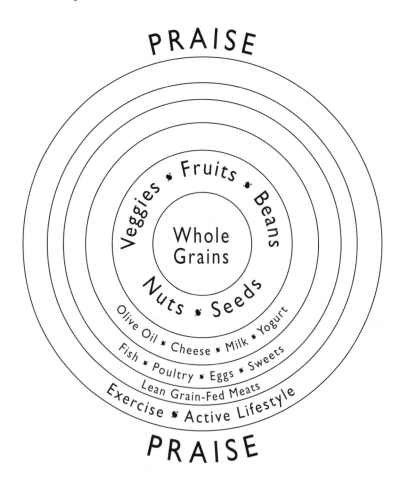

PRAISE

Veggies • Fruits • Beans
Whole Grains
Nuts • Seeds
Olive Oil • Cheese • Milk • Yogurt
Fish • Poultry • Eggs • Sweets
Lean Grain-Fed Meats
Exercise • Active Lifestyle

PRAISE

Go with the Grain

> *"Also take for yourself wheat, barley, beans, lentils, millet, and spelt; put them into one vessel, and make bread of them for yourself"* (Ezekiel 4:9).

Whole grains (whole wheat, brown or wild rice, barley, bulgur wheat, kasha, cornmeal, sprouted grain breads such as Ezekiel 4:9™, cereals, and pastas) make up the core. Ezekiel 4:9 brand and other *sprouted* grain breads are available at most health food stores.

Processed whole grain breads are also fine. Just make sure the bread you buy is not "enriched" wheat bread. Even if the bread is brown in color, it may be little more than spongy processed white bread with molasses in it to give it a brown color. What a disservice was done to us when "unnecessary" fiber and nutrients were processed out of bread to give us that melt-in-your-mouth fluff called white bread. Who wants bread to melt in their mouth? Vitamins and minerals are then shot back into the bread so it can be called "enriched." Does that make sense to you?

As mentioned in the previous chapter, if you have problems with digestion and suspect you have food sensitivities, try going without grain products (except for brown rice), dairy, soy, artificial sweeteners, and MSG for a month, and see what differences you notice in your digestion. Many have discovered that going without grains and foods with yeast in them have helped weight loss.

The Fruit (and Veggie) of the Land

> *"And God said, 'See, I have given you every herb that yields seed which is on the face of all the earth, and every tree whose fruit yields seed; to you it shall be for food'"* (Genesis 1:29).

God made man an omnivore, able to eat both plant and animal food, but He designed us to eat primarily grains and plant proteins. Our teeth and digestive system are different from a carnivore's. The majority of the teeth God gave us are perfect for grinding plant foods instead of ripping and tearing like a carnivore's teeth. Our long intestinal tract is made for the digestion of plant foods. Your dog, however, has a very short intestinal tract and has considerably more hydrochloric acid in his stomach than an herbivore or omnivore. The carnivore digests meat quickly and waste is eliminated soon after so it doesn't putrefy in a long intestinal tract.

Our second most important ring around the Food Circle represents vegetables, fruits, nuts, and seeds (including raw almonds, walnuts, sesame seeds, and sunflower seeds) and legumes (black beans, navy, pinto or kidney beans, split or black-eyed peas, chickpeas, lentils, and soybeans). Add nuts, seeds, and beans to salads and cooked vegetables for variety and flavor.

USDA's Recommended Daily Servings of Vegetables and Fruits

- three vegetables and two fruits for children ages two to six, less active women, and older adults
- four vegetables and three fruits for children over six, teenage girls, active women, and most men
- five vegetables and four fruits for teenage boys and active men

If you have a teenage son or active husband who is eating nine servings of fruits and vegetables a day, you deserve a gold star and an unlimited shopping spree at the department store of your choice!

When Paul and I met in 1987, he thought white pasta was the only food group. Actually, he would have been happy eating pasta every night. Knowing that pasta is…well, *paste* (remember making glue out of flour and water in school?), this dewy-eyed bride managed to introduce her groom to brown rice, whole wheat pasta, and big veggie salads. Over the years we've managed to move from spaghetti every day to once a week (twice a week if I'm out of town and the Pasta Prince has his way). So, if your husband or children think ketchup and fries constitute two servings of vegetables and Twinkies are a major food group, take heart. It's never too late to begin substituting more nutritious foods bit by bit.

How Big Is a Serving?

Thanks to biggie-sized servings and "all you can possibly eat until you fall over" buffets, we have a very distorted view of what constitutes a serving size. Most of us think in terms of platefuls, when actually a serving is closer to a small handful. I don't mean a Goliath-sized handful either. Think more in terms of David—or Ruth.

In January 2005, the USDA released their new dietary guidelines. They recommend two cups of fruit per day and two and a half cups of vegetables per day for most people.

Eating the recommended five to nine servings is simpler than you think. Here's an example of a day's worth of fruits and veggies:

- Breakfast: Small banana *or* ½ cup sliced strawberries (counts as one); add to cereal and milk (or add to BASIC Power Shake)
- Snack: ¼ cup of raisins (counts as one)
- Lunch: Salad with two cups of veggies (counts as two); mix with crumbled egg, croutons; one slice whole grain bread with butter
- Snack: Apple (counts as one) with one tablespoon almond or natural peanut butter
- Dinner: Small salad (counts as one) with one tablespoon dressing; chicken and brown rice with ½ cup green beans (counts as one)
- Grand total: Three fruit servings and four vegetable servings equal seven servings.

Time for an Oil Change?

> *"For the* Lord *your God is bringing you into a good land, a land of brooks of water, of fountains and springs, that flow out of valleys and hills; a land of wheat and barley, of vines and fig trees and pomegranates, a land of olive oil and honey"* (Deuteronomy 8:7-8).

The third ring is olive oil, cheese, milk, and yogurt. You may use any monounsaturated oil such as olive, almond, avocado, and peanut oils. Cold-pressed flaxseed oil is a rich source of omega-3 essential fatty acids, and organic coconut oil is rich in medium chain triglycerides. Unlike olive oil, it's tasteless, so you may use it for cooking and baking.

In Mediterranean cultures, olive oil is used in place of butter or shortening. Try putting a little in a small jar in the refrigerator and using it like butter. Mix flaxseed or olive oil with some apple cider vinegar or balsamic vinegar for an inexpensive, tasty, and healthful salad dressing.

Eating Her Curds and Whey

Use small amounts of pure butter, milk (raw and organic from cows that are free from antibiotic and hormone injections; or almond, rice, or soy milk), cheeses (parmesan, part skim mozzarella, feta, or cheese made from soy, rice, or almonds), yogurt (plain, skim, or low-fat; add fresh fruit and a little honey, or stevia leaf herbal sweetener). Avoid highly processed dairy products as much as possible.

Or If He Asks for a Fish...

> *"Then, as soon as they had come to land, they saw a fire of coals there, and fish laid on it, and bread.... Jesus then came and took the bread and gave it to them, and likewise the fish"* (John 21:9,13).

Jesus considered bread, fish, and eggs "good gifts" in Luke 11:11-13: "If a son asks for bread from any father among you, will he give him a stone? Or if he asks for a fish, will he give him a serpent instead of a fish? Or if he asks for an egg, will he offer him a scorpion? If you then, being evil [natural, carnal], know how to give good gifts to your children, how much more will your heavenly Father give the Holy Spirit to those who ask Him!"

A small amount of fish, poultry, eggs, and sweets makes up the fourth ring of our circle. Again, getting food as close to "God-made" as possible is best. In the Bible, fish with scales and fins are considered clean. Unclean are the scavengers such as catfish, crabs, and lobsters (which some nutritionists call "ocean cockroaches"). Look for cage-free poultry and their eggs, which are without antibiotics or growth hormones.

But what about cholesterol? Studies show that the yolk of the egg has the largest amount of cholesterol, but it also contains lecithin, which breaks the cholesterol down. In studies done at the University of Missouri, 70 people ate three eggs a day over a three-month period. Their blood tests showed an elevation of the "good" cholesterol (high density), and their triglyceride levels remained unchanged.[2]

Honey is also a good gift—in moderation. Honey is loaded with nutrients and enzymes. Just don't overdo it because honey is highly caloric, and too much of a good thing.... Well, why don't I let King Solomon tell you? Solomon was the wisest and richest man of his time. He wrote in Proverbs under the inspiration of God, "Have you found honey? Eat only as much as you need, lest you be filled with it and vomit" (Proverbs 25:16).

Little Stevia Wonder—Sweet and Good for You Too!

This little herb (related to the chrysanthemum family) may be the answer to our sugar and artificial sweetener woes. Studies on the dangers of sugar, corn syrup, and synthetic sweeteners are alarming.

Weight loss? Well, that's why we buy artificial sweeteners, right? According to some studies, however, artificial sweeteners may actually *stimulate* the appetite!

Good news! The leaves of a bushy little plant in Paraguay have been used for over 1500 years by South Americans to sweeten beverages and other foods.

Stevia comes in packets like sugar or in liquid and is available in health food stores. You should also find stevia cookbooks there. Not all stevia tastes the same, so ask your health food store owners which one they recommend. Some taste like sugar (such as Stevita and SweetLeaf) while others have a slight licorice taste.

Another natural sweetener that's gaining popularity is agave, from the juice of the agave cactus. It's a slow-releasing carbohydrate sweetener that looks and tastes like honey but with half the calories of sugar. While honey rates a 75 on the glycemic index (meaning it can really spike blood sugar), agave enters the bloodstream more slowly and registers a low 11, making it more acceptable for diabetics and those of us interested in weight control.

Is It Your Birthday? Okay, Have a Steak

> "And he said to him, 'Your brother has come, and because he has received him safe and sound, your father has killed the fatted calf'" (Luke 15:27).

In Jesus' day as well as in many Mediterranean cultures today, eating meat (beef, lamb, and veal) is reserved for special occasions only. As you can imagine, the cattle in biblical times were not subjected to living in overcrowded feedlots, fed moldy grain, or injected with antibiotics, growth hormones, and steroids as are today's cattle. Nutritionists have written much about the dangers of eating red meat—more than I could possibly cover in this section. If you are interested in learning more, I recommend Dr. Don Colbert's book

What Would Jesus Eat? In chapter 4, "The Meats That Jesus Ate," he discusses the benefits of eating grass-fed free-range cattle, the diseases associated with red meat, and the value of the biblical slaughter of animals versus the horrors of today's feedlots and slaughterhouses.[3] It's for neither the fainthearted nor those who would prefer to think hamburgers grow on trees.

Following our Mediterranean model, I do not recommend eating red meat every day. Fish, poultry, and eggs are the preferred animal foods. In Jesus' day, people killed the fatted calf on rare celebratory occasions, not daily. The people of the Bible would be astonished to find we have entire eating establishments dedicated to the eating of red meat—from steak houses to fast-food hamburger joints. If you do eat beef, look for grass-fed cattle, which have considerably less fat, toxins, and growth hormones than grain-fed feedlot cattle have.

Under the Old Covenant, pigs were unclean animals, and I do not recommend eating pork. You probably like ham, hot dogs, bacon, and other processed meats made from pork, but here's some information that may turn your head away from "the other white meat," as the National Pork Board calls it.

And This Little Piggie Went Wee-Wee-Wee All the Way Off the Cliff

Jesus, being a devout Jew, did not eat pork. In fact, He used pigs as receptacles for the demons within the Gadarene demoniac (Luke 8:26-39). The pigs were destroyed when they plunged off a cliff into the lake and drowned.

God didn't arbitrarily forbid the Jews from eating certain foods. Every meat God deemed unclean is unfit for human consumption. In 1953, science caught up with that truth when Dr. David Macht of Johns Hopkins University published a study on the toxicity of animals listed as clean and unclean in Leviticus 11 and Deuteronomy 14. He ran tests to determine their toxic effects on a controlled growth culture in his laboratory.[4]

Not surprisingly, every animal God calls toxic, science finds toxic too. Unclean animals include swine, horse, rabbit, squirrel, dog, cat, bear, opossum, groundhog, and rat. The clean animals (having cloven hooves and chewing the cud) include cattle, goats, sheep, oxen, and deer. Interestingly, the blood of all animals is more toxic than the flesh. God commands us not to eat the blood of animals.[5]

Many of the animals God calls unclean eat flesh or have parasites that would sicken or kill humans. Pigs, bears, and vultures eat decaying flesh. Wolves, lions, and other predators often prey on the weakest, sickliest animals in a herd.

Clean birds include poultry (chicken, turkey, geese), ducks, pigeons, and quail. Many supermarkets now carry chicken raised without antibiotics or hormones such as the MBA Brand Smart Chicken. We certainly don't need to be ingesting synthetic estrogen (a hormone typically given to chickens). Premenopausal, perimenopausal, and menopausal women need to be especially aware that hormonal imbalances may be linked to synthetic estrogen and estrogen-producing foods.

Instead of pork, how about turkey franks or kosher beef hot dogs once in a while? Many good soy products are available now from soy sausages and burgers to taco "meat" and chili. A stir-fry with fresh vegetables, crumbled soy burger, slivered almonds, and water chestnuts is a quick and easy dinner your family will love. If you're concerned about estrogen-producing foods, try fermented soy products such as tempeh instead of regular soy.

Fish—Clean and Unclean

The clean fish are those with scales and fins, including bass, tuna, salmon, trout, halibut, haddock, flounder, shad, perch, and sturgeon. Unclean aquatic animals are those without scales and fins: catfish, lobster, oysters, mussels, octopus, scallops, squid, shrimp, shark, clams, and crabs. Crustaceans such as lobsters and crabs are bottom dwellers that scavenge for dead animals on the sea floor. Similarly, shellfish such as clams, mussels, and oysters consume decaying organic matter and sewage that sinks to the sea floor.

Where I live, it's considered almost un-American *not* to eat catfish. Entire restaurants are dedicated to serving catfish (mostly fried). Although most catfish are raised in freshwater tanks, God created them to be purifiers of streams and lakes. The water in these tanks is most likely not pollutant-free, so contaminants are being passed on to the humans who eat them.

Archeological Evidence of the Benefits of Eating Clean

Archeological evidence suggests that the ancient Israelites were healthier than their Egyptian counterparts. In 1991 Jane Cahill published an article in the *Biblical Archeological Review* based on examinations she made of the remains of toilets in ancient Jewish, Roman, and Egyptian households. Jane must have a wry sense of humor because the article is entitled "It Had to Happen, Scientist Examines Ancient Bathrooms of Romans 568 B.C."

The Egyptian toilet remains showed evidence of eggs from tapeworms, trichinae, schistosomes, and wire worms (all found in pork). The remains of the Jewish toilets showed no parasites or infectious elements, only pollen from the vegetables, herbs, and fruits they had eaten.[6] In short: Eat clean, eat lean, and *always* eat green (lots of veggies!).

Servings 'Round the Food Circle

These are the recommended sizes of one serving of each item in the Food Circle:

- whole grains—1 slice whole grain bread; 1 ounce ready-to-eat cereal; ½ cup cooked cereal, rice, or pasta

- vegetables and fruit—1 medium-sized fruit; 1 cup of raw leafy vegetables; ½ cup chopped raw vegetables; ½ cup cut-up fruit; ½ cup frozen or cooked fruit or vegetables; ¾ cup (6 ounces) 100 percent juice; ¼ cup dried fruit

- legumes, nuts, and seeds—½ cup cooked or canned legumes (peas or beans); 10 almonds; 1 tablespoon seeds; 2 tablespoons almond butter or other nut butter

- olive oil, cheese, milk, yogurt—1–2 teaspoons olive oil; 1½ ounces cheese; 1 cup milk or yogurt

- fish, poultry, eggs, sweets—2–3 ounces cooked fish or poultry; 2 eggs (or egg whites); 1 teaspoon honey

- meats—2–3 ounces cooked lean meat, preferably free-range

Success Strategy #2

Tummy Curfew: The Quickest Way to Win at Losing

One of the most effective tools to aid weight loss and to improve sleep, digestion, and overall well-being is to stop eating three hours before bedtime. If your body is still digesting food while you sleep, you're not getting the rest you need to fully recover and firm up the lean muscle you're building by working out and eating the right foods. You also don't have much of an opportunity to burn off those calories you ate, so guess where they go? Ummm...the Fat Fairy makes it all go away? Nooooo. How about your hips and thighs?

If you're like me, you may have eaten a good, healthy diet during the day but heard the refrigerator calling your name at night. Have you ever stood in front of the refrigerator and just stared? I'd wake up half a gallon of something later and wonder how I got there.

Nighttime Food Cravings

Late-night eating is a common problem and a major cause of weight gain. Studies show that overweight people tend to eat most of their calories later in the day, while people at their normal weight tend to eat more calories earlier in the day.

"Fueling the Furnace" (eating smaller amounts every three to four hours) and eating a good breakfast so you won't overeat later in the day are two *physical* things you can do now to take control over late-night eating. But what about when those cravings hit? What else can you do?

Sowing to the Spirit

> *"Do not be deceived, God is not mocked; for whatever a man sows, that he will also reap. For he who sows to his flesh will of the flesh reap corruption, but he who sows to the Spirit will of the Spirit reap everlasting life"* (Galatians 6:7-8).

When is your toughest time? After 7:00 P.M.? After 9:00 P.M.? All day? Regardless of what time is hardest for you, I'd like you to take a 30- to 60-minute period during that tricky time and sow a seed of discipline to the Spirit.

What does that mean? You can choose to operate in the fruit of the Spirit within you at any time. As the phrase implies, the fruit of the Spirit is a gift from God and not something we have to drum up our-selves. One way to strengthen and cultivate the development of the fruit of self-control, for example, is to choose to accomplish some-thing that requires you to exercise self-control. You *yield* to the Holy Spirit within you and to His ability to operate in self-control. It's *His* fruit after all, so He knows how to use it. By choosing to do this activity, you are sowing a seed to the Spirit, and as we've just read, "He who sows to the Spirit will of the Spirit reap everlasting life."

The more seeds of self-control you sow to the Spirit and the more you yield to the ability of the Holy Spirit within you, the stronger the fruit of self-control becomes. By choosing to yield to the other eight fruit of the Spirit (love, joy, peace, patience, kindness, goodness, faithfulness, and gentleness), you will walk more and more in the Spirit "and you shall not fulfill the lust of the flesh."[7]

Why is the fruit of self-control so important? Self-control, also known as restraint or temperance, protects you from the enemy like the thick walls of a city protected it from invasion. "Like a city whose walls are broken down is a man who lacks self-control" (Proverbs 25:28 NIV). A life without restraint is not freedom—it's bondage to every whim of the flesh and temptation of the enemy. Like the inhabitants of a fortified city, the hearts of those whose lives are fortified by the fruit of self-control experience peace.

Here's the Plan

If your biggest temptation time is after 7:00 P.M., would you be willing to sow a seed of discipline and self-control from 7:00 to 8:00 P.M.? If you've already had your dinner, all I'm asking you to do is not to eat from 7:00 to 8:00 P.M. We'll start there. Commit this time to the Lord and let Him know you want to develop the fruit of self-control during this time. It would also be helpful for you to choose to operate in the fruit of patience (or patient endurance) and faithfulness—show up and refuse to give up!

Whatever activity you choose, do it "as to the Lord." The benefits? Supernatural! "Whatever you do, do it heartily, as to the Lord and not to men, knowing that from the Lord you will receive the reward of the inheritance; for you serve the Lord Christ."[8] That thrills me! You will receive the reward of the inheritance from the Lord! When you sow a seed of the fruit of self-control *to* the Spirit, you will reap life *from* the Spirit. What you sow, you will reap. When you plant seeds of self-control, you will have strength in areas where you had little or no control before. Determine to sow in faith to the Spirit and you *will* reap (absolutely, definitely, and positively!). Remember that the secret of your success is not some diet but the development of the fruit of the Spirit, which becomes part of your sanctified lifestyle.

In faith, you can plant seeds of self-control, faithfulness, and patient endurance to the Lord, and you will be rewarded with increase in that area. And though fruit doesn't ripen overnight, it does develop and mature.

When a farmer plants seeds and waters them, what does he harvest? Seeds? No! Crops—big, beautiful, abundant crops from the teeny-tiny little seeds he planted. So what can you expect to reap from these good seeds you sow? That's right—the good fruit of the seeds you've planted. God is faithful.

Seeds to Sow

Whether your most vulnerable time to overeat is in the morning, afternoon, or evening, here are some activities you can do today in faith. Choose one or combine several. Speak to your heavenly Father and let Him know you are sowing a seed of self-control to the Spirit by choosing to do this activity "as to the Lord" instead of eating.

1. Read through, sign, and date the Step-UP Commitment in chapter 10.

2. Take a walk by yourself or with the family.

3. Do a PraiseMoves workout (chapter 9) or other workout video or DVD.

4. Brush your teeth—and I don't mean casually either. Brush, floss, brush again, use mouthwash, and rinse. Get tooth whitening trays, add the whitening solution, and wear them for 30 to 60 minutes. If you're thirsty, you can still drink water through a straw.

5. Clean out and reorganize one or two dresser drawers.

6. File into a neat organizer those business cards you've collected.

7. Go through the mail that's stacked up on your desk.

8. Write the thank-you note you've been intending to write.

9. Shoot some hoops or play catch or badminton with the kids.

10. Give the dog a bath. Don't have a dog? Give the kids a bath. Better yet, get some candles, soft music, and a good book, and take a long, relaxing bath yourself!

11. Go through *one section* of your closet and take out everything you've not worn in more than a year. Unless it's a costume for a play you intend to do in the near future, get rid of any old, torn, too small, or too large clothing. Put the clothes in a box or bag and put them where you can give them away to a mission or Goodwill tomorrow. And don't just give away the old, worn-out things. Think of the person receiving it. Put a few nice things in there that you may or may not be wearing now. Do it just because you want to bless someone with something nice. Pray over the clothing, that the recipients will be drawn closer to the Lord. The fun thing is that you may consider the nice clothes you're giving away to be a seed you're planting for nice new clothes for you—a fit new you too! Remember, "He who sows sparingly will also reap sparingly, and he who sows bountifully will also reap bountifully."[9]

12. Write a get-well or "I've been thinking about you" card to a friend or relative. E-mails are great, but there's nothing like realizing someone took the time, love, and care to actually write out a physical card and mail it.

13. Sew (not sow!) that button or mend that tear that's been keeping you from wearing a favorite blouse or pair of slacks.

14. Write a prayer to the Lord in your journal (or note-book).

15. Write down three miracles you want to see happen in your life. Miracles are God's specialty, you know!

16. Look through your bookshelves and take out books you can give to the church or public library. If you've finished reading them and really don't want them anymore, why not let someone else enjoy them? If your church doesn't have a lending library, your books could be the start of one!

17. Read an uplifting Christian book or classic and sip water with a slice of lemon.

18. Pray for persecuted Christians and for missionaries on the foreign field and the people they are reaching with the gospel.

19. Pray for our president and leaders in government, the school board and teachers, your pastor and those in ministry at your church and in other churches, women and children in need, and the lost in your community.

20. Sing a song of praise to the Lord. Sing a new song if you'd like—one that comes right out of your heart to Him!

A BASIC (Body And Soul In Christ) Step

By choosing to do something constructive when you have an urge to eat, you are accomplishing several things at once.

- "Body": Physically, you are involved in an activity other than eating.

- "Soul" (your mind, will, and emotions): You are exercising control over your feelings by choosing to respond to them differently. You can decide not to eat when you experience cravings and choose to do something else instead.

- "In Christ": You are sowing seeds of self-control, faithfulness, and patient endurance by yielding to the fruit of the Spirit. You are choosing to do this "as to the Lord," thus sowing to the Spirit with a capital *S*.

A BASIC Step involves all of you: your spirit, soul, and body.

You are also eliminating a major stress maker in your life. All those little things that get left undone because you haven't taken the time to do them have been nagging at the back of your mind. "All or nothing" thinking has convinced us that if we don't have time to complete a project perfectly from start to finish in one sitting, we shouldn't even try to begin. Now you're taking control and relieving stress by choosing to organize a small section of your closet, selecting to rearrange your sock drawer instead of all the drawers, or taking a ten-minute walk with the family instead of thinking, *One day we'll climb Mt. Everest....*

Lastly, you've just given yourself another reason to praise the Lord and yes, feel good about yourself too. You can decide that the "I have to eat something" signal means "I'm going to exercise now," or "I'll see if the kids want to play a board game," or "Who was I going to call, write to, or visit?" Have you ever given in to eating when you were *avoiding* doing something else? I have. Ask yourself, *What am I trying to avoid doing?* You don't have to be a slave to temptation any longer. You can then wholeheartedly say, "You know what? I can do all things through Christ who strengthens me!"[10]

Success Strategy #3

God's Heavenly Weigh: Garnish Your Plate with Praise

Most of us are accustomed to thanking God for our meal before we start eating. I propose that we encircle our dining experience with praise.

In Isaiah 55:2 the Lord says, "Listen carefully to Me, and eat what is good, and let your soul delight itself in abundance."

Do you see the three parts of that Scripture?

1. "Listen carefully to Me."
2. "Eat what is good."
3. "Let your soul delight itself in abundance."

Not long ago I was prayer journaling. (That involves writing prayers to God and recording what you believe He is telling you in the Scriptures and in your heart.) I wrote, "Father, how can I best reach and maintain the healthy ideal weight and size for me?" The idea (or revelation) that occurred to me was so complete and made so much sense that I must have stopped and stared for a full minute in wide-eyed wonder.

The Lord led me to Isaiah 55:2 and this plan: Give the Lord a portion of your food every day. How? Since you can't physically give that food to the Lord, substitute it with praise and thanksgiving. Your portion is the food you eat. The portion you give to the Lord is your offering of praise and thanksgiving. The physical food you leave on the plate serves as a symbol of the sacrifice of praise you will be offering Him from your heart.

Take a quick look back at the graphic of the Food Circle under Success Strategy #1. See how it's surrounded by a ring of praise? That's the ideal.

You know how "full" you feel when you completely throw yourself into praise and worship? Or if that's not your style, can you recall a time when you were so tremendously thankful for an answered prayer or the Lord's intervention at the exact moment you needed Him most that you thought you'd burst? That's what I mean.

I used to eat way past the point of satisfying my physical hunger to fill a void of a different kind. Have you done that? If you will eat *slowly* enough to be sensitive to when your stomach is satisfied, you will recognize when to stop eating—even if there's still food on your plate. Put your fork down, and if you're alone, start praising the Lord. Thank Him for who He is in your life. Worship Him for His amazing attributes and His love for you. You and God will enjoy a time of sweet communion. After all, He is the "bread of life" that truly satisfies. You may be amazed at how quickly you feel satisfied.

If you are with the family or out to dinner at a restaurant, when you sense that you are no longer hungry, put your fork down and silently praise and worship the Lord. Thank Him in your heart. You don't have to be flaky about it. No need to be rude or hyper-spiritual and shut everyone else out because you're communing with God. Hoo-wee, what a witness!

Instead, why not tell those at your table something wonderful the Lord has done for you or someone you know? In the Psalms, David often spoke of telling others about the Lord's marvelous works. That's praising Him! No one has to know what you're doing if you don't want them to know. It's a great opportunity to tell your children why you love and trust in the Lord. Share an experience of what God did for you, for someone in your family, or for someone in the Bible. You might begin by saying, "I was thinking about how much the Lord loves us." You'll be giving glory to God and "satisfying your soul with abundance" at the same time.

What If You Don't Have a "Full Signal"?

You may be like I was. I had spent so many years overeating and using food to stuff down emotional pain that I really didn't know when I was hungry or when I had had enough. All I knew was I could not control myself around food. I saw food and I wanted to eat it, and I would eat it until either my stomach hurt or I drugged myself to sleep. Not a pretty picture.

When I came to Christ, I found out that nothing was too small to ask Him about. As long as I could find something in His Word to confirm my prayers, I could ask. I found 3 John 2: "Beloved, I pray that you may prosper in all things and be in health, just as your soul prospers." Compulsive overeating was not my idea of being "in health," so I asked the Lord to heal me. I asked Him to give me the ability to know when I'd eaten enough food and the desire to stop once I'd had enough.

I will never forget the moment I experienced the "full response" for the first time since I was six years old. I was a newlywed. Paul and I were sitting at our little dining room table at dinner. Toward the end of the meal, I felt as if something gently dropped and expanded slightly in my stomach. It was the last little bit of food that tipped the scales from "not full" to "full." I felt it! For the first time in more than 20 years I felt I had enough food without feeling stuffed or using tremendous willpower to stop eating.

"I just felt my full signal!" I practically shouted to Paul across the table from me. "Your what?" he asked. How could he know what I was talking about? He patiently listened as I explained it, tears in my eyes. Paul realized I just had a breakthrough even though he didn't fully understand. (He is the kind of person who can eat a third of a piece of candy, wrap up the remaining two thirds, and put it away for another day. Amazing.)

Ask God to restore the natural "full signal" response for you again. I'm often reminded, "You do not have because you do not ask."[11]

Eat in Faith

> *"But he who doubts is condemned if he eats, because he does not eat from faith; for whatever is not from faith is sin"* (Romans 14:23).

If you have not experienced the "full signal" in more years than you can remember, or if you are unsure if you can leave food on your plate, take heart. Determine to walk out your healing by faith, practice "God's Heavenly Weigh," and garnish your plate with praise. Prepare your food with an eye to portion control (see portion sizes at the end of "Success Strategy #1"). Eat slowly and stop eating when you still have some food on your plate. Put your fork down and praise the Lord for your healing, your deliverance, for who He is to you, and for every other wonderful thing about Him that comes to you.

Don't wait until you feel like praising God. It probably won't happen. Like everything else God commands, it's done by faith. Faith is believing and acting with the calm assurance that the Word of God is true—regardless of how we feel. Bible-based faith is more powerful than feeling or seeing—it's believing God.

Success Strategy #4

Vitamins and Dietary Supplements—Just Nice, or Necessary?

Since we are striving to eat foods as close to the way God made them as possible, why do we need to take vitamins and other dietary supplements? Vitamins tablets aren't exactly as God made them, are they? Here we seem to have a dilemma. No, vitamin tablets and capsules do not grow on trees; however, the vast majority of nutritionists and dieticians as well as many doctors now advocate the use of high-quality vitamins and dietary supplements.

The *Journal of the American Medical Association (JAMA)* made big news on June 19, 2002, when it reversed its long-standing decision that taking vitamin supplements was unnecessary. In a scientific review article by R.H. Fletcher, M.D., and K.M. Fairfeld, M.D., the researchers advised doctors that the use of vitamin supplements is wise in the fight against many chronic degenerative diseases.[12] "It appears prudent for all adults to take vitamin supplements," they stated.

JAMA's pronouncement seems to reflect the adage spoken by America's revered inventor Thomas Edison: "The doctor of the future will give no medicine, but will interest his patients in the care of the human body, in diet, and in the cause and prevention of disease."

We want to stress that vitamins, minerals, and herbs are called *supplements* for a reason. They are meant to supplement, or complement, a healthy diet. Nutritional supplements are not a substitute for good, quality foods. It would be ludicrous to live on Cokes and French fries and then pop some vitamin pills and expect to be healthy.

When choosing supplements, go for quality. A dietary supplement that does what it says it will do and makes a difference for you is worth 20 cheapies that are little more than wimpy sugar pills!

A sign at a local health store reads, "You think health is expensive? Try sickness."

Why Nutritional Supplements?

We already know the important role a good diet plays in the quality of our health. Why can't we just get all the nutrition we need from the food we eat?

Over the years the quality of our food supply has changed. Our ancestors ate lots of unprocessed, nutrient-dense foods grown in mineral-rich soil. Cooking and industrialized processing of foods causes nutrients to be lost. That's why I recommend several servings of fresh, raw vegetables and fruits every day.

Considering the *quality* of food has changed, to receive the same amount of nutrients our ancestors received we would have to greatly increase the *quantity* of foods we eat daily. Here we seem to be in a quandary. Most of us are already eating too much for our sedentary lifestyles. Our ancestors were much more active than the average man or woman in North America today. Not surprisingly, they were able to eat heaping helpings of food and not gain weight. Everyday life was a prolonged aerobic workout! For example, the 132-pound woman of today who works in an office setting burns about 720 calories of energy during an eight-hour workday. By comparison, our ancestors a few thousand years ago burned 2160 calories working and gathering food for their families over the same period of time.[13]

The Essentials

The foundation of any supplementation program should be a good *multivitamin* containing at least 400 micrograms of the B vitamin folic acid. Folic acid is essential for women of childbearing age.

To build and retain strong bones, bodies of all ages need *calcium*. Most people don't get enough calcium from their diets. The Food and

Nutrition Board of the Institute of Medicine says everyone over eight years of age needs at least 1000 milligrams of calcium per day. Teens and senior citizens need more—between 1200 to 1300 milligrams.

We've discussed the havoc oxidative stress can have on the body. *Antioxidant vitamins* E and C may help protect against conditions linked to oxidative damage, such as heart disease, cancer, and cataracts. The recommended dietary allowance for vitamin C is only 60 to 90 milligrams per day, but many who regularly supplement vitamin C take between 250 and 1000 milligrams per day. In clinical studies, vitamin C supplementation at levels at or above 1000 milligrams per day has regularly lowered the incidence and duration of the common cold.[14]

Vitamin E is a powerful antioxidant said to reduce the risk of cardiovascular disease, boost immune system function, reduce cancer risk, and work topically as an agent in wound healing. The RDA for vitamin E is 30 IU (International Units), but most research studies indicate 100 to 800 IU will yield greater health benefits. Eating that much vitamin E in our food daily is not possible, so additional supplementation is needed.

Essential fatty acids, as the name implies, are essential to our health—and most people are horribly deficient in them. Our bodies cannot manufacture EFAs. They help the body produce hormones and are important in cardiovascular health and cholesterol regulation, and they contain anti-inflammatory compounds that relieve arthritis and autoimmune diseases. They provide necessary building blocks for healthy body structure and provide an important source of energy for cells. If you have dry skin, are losing hair, and feel cold all the time, you may be deficient in essential fatty acids.

Many nutritionists recommend taking one to two tablespoons of flaxseed oil daily, which is rich in EFAs. Adding it to salads or a BASIC Power Shake makes that easy. Fish oils in capsule form (600 to 1200 milligrams daily) are another way to ensure you're getting the EFAs your body needs. If you prefer to take your EFAs in fish oil capsule form and you have a sensitive stomach, I recommend taking them with a meal to keep from experiencing the dreaded "fishy burp."

Special Needs

Some supplements are specifically designed to assist with vision, menopause, sports performance, memory, arthritis, mild depression, prostate health, and more. Again, speak with a health care professional who is up-to-date on the latest advancements in nutraceuticals, phytochemicals, and dietary supplementation.

Glyconutrients: The Missing Links?

An exciting and recent discovery in the world of nutritional supplementation is the group called *glyconutrients*. *Glyco* means "sweet," but these simple sugars are very different from ordinary table sugar. They appear to be the "missing links" that supply the building blocks for healthy cells and make possible accurate cell-to-cell communication.

How does your body know to heal itself when you get a paper cut? How does your digestive tract differentiate between nutrients it needs for cellular health and those it should expel? How does your body deal with toxins? The answers lie in the glycoform messages formed by these dietary sugars, which enable cells to communicate with each other.

This science is so new that no papers in English appeared on the subject in the 1960s, yet now thousands of scientific papers are being written on them every year (more than 20,000 glycoscience publications in 1998 alone!).[15]

Five of these essential sugars appear in human breast milk. They seem to play an important role in immune system and hormonal function. Potential health benefits include tissue healing; positive effects on asthma, rheumatoid arthritis, and lupus; arthritis prevention and reduced pain in joint mobility; improvement in diabetes; and protection against stress-related illnesses. Glyconutrients may relieve symptoms of fibromyalgia, chronic fatigue syndrome, and ADHD. They may even inhibit cancerous tumor growth and tumor cell metastasis.[16]

For additional information on this fascinating new realm of scientific study, I suggest you read some of the educational and scientific articles available at www.GlycoScience.org or look at some other resources listed at www.BasicSteps.info.

Get Some Green Powdered Stuff

Whether it's powdered spirulina, kamut grass, wheat grass, barley grass, chlorella, spinach, quinoa sprouts, green tea, or all of it combined—get some powdered green stuff and add it to your BASIC Power Shake every morning. These super green foods provide phytonutrients and other potent antioxidants that help protect the body from free radical damage. They also help detoxify and nourish the body.

Since we often cannot get the amounts of fresh fruits and vegetables we'd like (and most likely we couldn't eat the appropriate amounts for optimal health), a container of these wonderful concentrated green foods can deliver the nutrition found in several servings of vegetables in one or two scoops.

For my personal recommendations and the latest information on nutritional supplementation and fitness, please visit www.Basic-Steps.info.

Bringing It Home

In this chapter, I learned this about…

the food circle:_____

_____

the tummy curfew:_____

_____

"God's Heavenly Weigh":_____

_____

vitamins and dietary supplements: _____

_____

I can start doing this better today: _____

_____

Lord, I ask You to help me _____

_____

4

Movement:
Are You Sitting Down?

Sitting down—that seems to be the great American pastime. I know of no other culture willing to pay so much for convenience.

We recently had a satellite system installed so we could get Sky Angel Christian programming. We live in the country, so we have no cable television and barely three network stations. The young men we hired to install the dish showed us all the wonderful things the satellite and remote control could do.

"Put this wire in your phone jack, and you'll be able to see who's calling you on the television screen without ever having to get up to look at the caller ID on your phone," said one of the young men.

I thought that caller ID was already a high-level convenience to keep me from having to answer the phone if I didn't want to answer it. Now another level of convenience was attainable. I didn't even have to get off the couch to look at the convenient caller ID if I preferred not to move the ten feet to the telephone.

"Yeah," said the other worker, smiling. "If I'm watching something on TV and the phone rings, I can see who's calling without even having to get up."

"Without even having to get up," I repeated, amazed.

"You want me to show you how?" he asked.

"No, thank you," I said. "That's more convenience than I can handle."

Sedentary—Sedative—Sedated

If you were to ask most fitness experts what one thing they considered most responsible for the obesity epidemic, they would probably say it was our sedentary lifestyle.

Sedentary, sedative, and *sedated* are three words that have a lot in common. They come from the same Latin root word *sedere,* meaning "to sit." Obviously, a sedentary lifestyle is characterized by much sitting. Sitting in one place long enough seems to act like a sedative, doesn't it? We don't want to move. The biggest impetus to move may come from the TV commercial urging us to raid the refrigerator.

Before I began exercising regularly, I led a very sedentary life. A couple of times a year I would become disgusted enough with myself to go on a health binge for a while. I'd exercise like a mad woman for a few days and then sink into the couch like Attila the Slug for the next three months.

My excuses? Too busy, no time, it's boring…and the all-time favorite, "I don't wanna!"

Again, God leads us to balance our lives. If we get too far on one side of the road or the other, we fall into a ditch.

Some are quick to say, "Yeah, but doesn't the Bible say 'Exercise profits little'?" Well, close. In his letter to Timothy, Paul recommended that Timothy train himself to be godly in character just as the athlete trains himself to be physically superior. He wrote, "For bodily exercise profits a little, but godliness, is profitable for all things."[1] One interpretation says exercise profits for "a little while." The Greeks of Paul's day held physical training in high esteem. Athletic events such as the Olympics were very important to them. Paul is telling us that while physical exercise may profit us in this life, it is not to be compared with godliness, which benefits us both here and eternally, "having promise of the life that now is and of that which is to come."[2]

Paul often compared the Christian life to the endurance and training of runners and boxers. He certainly was not against physical exercise. It just wasn't a priority to him. We must also realize that life during Bible times was considerably more arduous than it is today. Paul and Silas didn't have to go down to Gold's Gym to pump some iron. Their day-to-day existence provided plenty of exercise. Those who followed additional exercise and strength-building regimens did so for sporting events, not because they needed to lose a few pounds.

Lives that expended so much energy for daily existence needed no additional physical exercise. It's no wonder physical fitness is not a big topic of discussion in the Scriptures. But Paul does tell us to "present your bodies a living sacrifice"[3] and treat our bodies well, for they are the "temple of the Holy Spirit."[4] We are responsible to be good stewards, or guardians, of our bodies. "You are not your own," Paul continues. "For you were bought at a price." That price was the shed blood of Jesus Christ. This is a cause for rejoicing! We can say, "My body belongs to the Lord. He knows how to fix it. He will help me get it in shape!"

Do I *Have to* Exercise?

No. You don't have to do anything. If you want to be healthy, however, you do have to *move*.

In July of 1996, the Office of the Surgeon General released the following statement: "The Surgeon General has determined that the lack of physical activity is detrimental to your health." The report also equated *not* exercising with smoking a pack of cigarettes a day!

I was excited to see exercise included in the USDA's 2005 dietary guidelines. (This is a first and reminds me of the food circle.) To reduce the risk of chronic disease in adulthood, participate in 30 minutes of moderate-intensity physical activity above your usual activity on most (or preferably every) day of the week. This could include walking at three and a half mph, stretching, light weight-lifting, or gardening.

To lose excess weight and prevent gradual, unhealthy weight gain as we age, the USDA recommends 60 minutes of daily moderate- to vigorous-intensity physical activity, such as walking at four and a half mph, aerobics, jogging, and swimming freestyle. To maintain weight loss however, the USDA recommends 60 to 90 minutes of *daily* moderate-intensity activity. Most people should consult their health care provider before beginning a moderate-intensity exercise program.

Many people would prefer completing their daily exercise in one or two sessions, but that's not always practical. Breaking some of your exercise into 10- or 15-minute segments on a busy day could be the difference between getting that workout accomplished and letting it slide for the day, which could lead to yet another day off....

You can choose to start living a more active lifestyle. *Activity* and *movement* may sound better to you than *exercise*. For many of us, *exercise* brings up unhappy school memories in baggy green gym clothes. I remember lying on the floor with the rest of the girls in gym class and flinging our hips and legs into the air doing the "bicycle" to the song "Go, You Chicken Fat, Go!" I was sure the other girls thought the song was about me.

If your memories of exercising are equally unglamorous or if you simply don't like to perspire or muss your hair, you may not be as happy to hear that to be healthy you must raise your heart rate and break a sweat by moving your body several times a week.

Like our spiritual condition, our physical health declines if we don't develop it. We may seem to be able to coast for a while—until a situation arises that calls for some muscle, and we fall back exhausted, unable to rise to the occasion.

On the Bright Side

We think of exercise as a mainly cosmetic fix, don't we? Women's magazines shout at us from the checkout line: "Get Bikini Thin in Only Minutes a Day!" "Rock-Hard Abs in Seconds!" "The Secret-Weapon Workout!"

The problem with that is that we can think, *Get real, girl. I'm never going to look like those models. Why bother exercising?*

Fitness is so much more than the circumference of your waist and thigh (thank goodness!). Here are just a few of the wonderful benefits we can derive from more physical activity:

- lowers risks for cancer, heart disease, and stroke
- lowers tension and reduces stress
- increases endurance, stamina, and flexibility
- promotes better sleep
- lowers blood pressure and cholesterol levels
- leads to healthier pregnancies
- improves mood and lowers risk of depression or anxiety
- decreases risk of osteoporosis
- lowers health care bills and lessens dependence on prescribed medications
- improves mental alertness and ability to concentrate
- improves sexual relations

- helps us look and feel younger and improves the complexion
- lowers risk of developing diabetes
- lowers insulin, allowing fat to leave the fat cells to be burned as fuel
- strengthens the immune system
- strengthens bones and joints, tones muscles, and increases lean body mass
- decreases appetite, raises metabolism, and increases calories burned

Plastic surgery is only skin deep, but exercise benefits us inside and out. Some encouraging news for those of us over 30 years old is that more mature women appear to gain the most benefits from exercise.

So Why Don't We Do It?

Our reasons for not purposefully adding more activity to our lives sound like the reasons we've given for not eating breakfast (although we're all doing that now, right?).

Perhaps the reason we put exercise off is that we value our excuses more than the reasons we need to exercise. What if you looked at eating food or bathing yourself the same way you looked at exercise? *I don't have time to eat this week. I think I'll wait until the first of the month to take a shower.* Seems pretty ridiculous, doesn't it?

Well, let's stop rationalizing and start realizing that exercise is as important to our overall well-being as eating healthy food and acquainting our bodies with soap at least once a day. What are some of the things you always put at the top of your list each day? These are the things that are such a part of your daily routine that you don't even have to write them down to remember to do them. Your job? Feeding the family? Prayer? Picking the children up from school or day care? Wearing clean clothes? Brushing your teeth?

You have probably also developed some good habits that aren't as vital as making sure your children are fed—things that make you feel better once you do them. These habits might include making the bed, hanging up clothes, fixing your hair, and putting on makeup. You might even feel something's missing if you leave the house without doing these little tasks. Exercise can become that sort of discipline.

Thomas Edison said, "Opportunity is missed by most people because it is dressed in overalls and looks like work." You have the opportunity to change the quality of the rest of your life by investing a few minutes a day in exercise.

The Saboteur Under Your Feet

A warning: Someone wants you to live an inactive, low-energy, unhealthy life and leave the earth before your time. One of the names of the devil is "the deceiver." He has no real power over Christians, so he delights in deceiving us to use our God-given power against ourselves. How? By using our thoughts and words.

Did you know that worry is meditating on the devil's plans, just as faith is meditating on God's plans? Things that we worry about have a way of creeping out of our mouths. I'm sure that's one of the reasons the Lord inspired Paul to write, "Whatever things are true, whatever things are noble, whatever things are just, whatever things are pure, whatever things are lovely, whatever things are of good report, if there is any virtue and if there is anything praiseworthy—meditate on these things."[5]

What does that have to do with exercise? Well, I know I certainly didn't feel like taking a walk whenever I've entertained thoughts such as, *Oh, what's the use? I'll always be fat. I'm so out of shape I couldn't lift an eyebrow. I think my get-up-and-go got up and went. I better just take a nap instead.* Those thoughts dictated my actions.

Were these God-inspired thoughts? Did Jesus want to bless me with thoughts like that? No! Well, where did they come from? We have a lot of old programming in our heads—"old tapes" we need to erase and reprogram with the Word of God. You also have an enemy who wants to frustrate your every good plan. When thoughts like that occur, we can say, "Hey! I don't think like that!" You can take out your sword of the Spirit (the Word of God)[6] and agree with what God has to say instead.

Positive affirmations that are not based on the Word of God have only limited effectiveness. Scriptural affirmations work because God's Word is powerful. Sure, you could say, "Every day, in every way, I'm getting better and better." But our words are much more effective when we affirm the Word of God by saying, "I can do all things through Christ who strengthens me. I am strong in the Lord and the power of His might. I'm more than a conqueror through Him who loves me!"[7]

Dwelling on negative thoughts is impossible when those God-inspired, faith-filled words come out of your mouth. Since God's words are "life to those who find them, and health to all their flesh,"[8] the more you dwell on God's words and thoughts, the healthier and stronger you'll become spiritually, emotionally, and physically.

Now that we've confronted obstacles to taking control of your physical fitness, let's look at some options.

Do I Have to Do Aerobics?

If you think of aerobics as a dance class led by an instructor, no, you don't have to do aerobics. To be healthy, however, you will have to do aerobic exercise. *Aerobic* means "with air or oxygen." Aerobic activity is relatively long in duration, rhythmic, and low in intensity. Aerobic activities include walking (outdoors or on a treadmill), bicycle riding, dancing, jogging, swimming, rebounding (bouncing on a mini-trampoline), cross-country skiing, working out at aerobic dance classes, or exercising to videos and DVDs.

Anaerobic means just the opposite. Anaerobic activities are short in duration and high in intensity, such as weight lifting, sprinting, racquetball, and football. Exercising anaerobically tires a person more quickly. We will be talking later about the importance of weight and resistance training in your overall fitness routine, but right now we'll focus on aerobic activity you can start today.

You should be able to carry on a short conversation while doing any aerobic activity. If you find yourself gasping for air while talking, slow down. You may be working anaerobically, meaning you will feel tired more quickly and may experience sore muscles after your workout.

For fat loss, some sources recommend brisk walking progressing to 45 minutes or more daily. The combination of aerobic and anaerobic exercise seems to burn more fat than either type of exercise alone. That's why I'm including some anaerobic lean muscle-building in the Gimme Ten Workout, which follows.

Exercise not only helps metabolize fat and burn calories, but also reduces food cravings for overeaters and for women who crave certain types of food prior to menstruation. Excercise helps stabilize blood sugar levels, tone muscles, and keep the skin more supple. If you exercise less than three times a week, you need to increase your level of physical activity.

A brisk 30- to 45-minute walk three to five times a week will burn off enough calories to lose a pound a week (or more) if you're also following the healthy eating guidelines outlined in *BASIC Steps*.

Please see your doctor for a good overall checkup before beginning an exercise program. You should know before you begin an exercise program whether you have any physical limitations. You can pay closer attention to building up these areas of weakness and praying about them to the Lord too. He will give you wisdom about it if you will ask Him.

The Lord gave a very practical, up-to-date message to us through the apostle James when he wrote, "If any of you lacks wisdom, let him ask of God, who gives to all liberally and without reproach, and it will be given to him."[9] I heard of a young lady who asked the Lord to be her personal trainer and help her restore her body to be the healthy, fit temple God intended it to be. What a great idea!

If you haven't been exercising on a regular basis, increase your physical activity gradually until your body becomes stronger and exercise is easier to do. Start with five or ten minutes of walking or rebounding, and after a week or two, add ten minutes to each workout. Get some muscle to help you become fit faster by following the Gimme Ten Workout.

Have a Plan—Have Two!

Six A.M. You're up! Ah—it's Monday morning, and you planned to begin your new workout program today. But the baby's crying, the dog ate your exercise DVD, and the electricity went out during the night—it's really 6:30 A.M., not 6:00. Should you throw your exercise plan out the window? No! Go to plan B.

What is plan B? That's the "divide it up" plan. One 30-minute workout becomes three 10-minute workouts during the day. Instead of the brisk 30-minute walk you'd planned, try this:

- Before breakfast do a Gimme Ten Workout for ten minutes.
- Before lunch, take a brisk walk for ten minutes.
- Before dinner, bounce on the rebounder or jog in place while watching the news for ten minutes.

By having alternatives to plan A, you ensure you will not have to hang your head in despair. We must guard against that sort of "all or nothing" thinking. God wants us to live our lives in balance. Don't give up just because the plan A exercise you thought you would do doesn't work today.

I was a great excuse maker. If something came up and I couldn't follow my food or exercise plan for the day, I'd throw all caution to the wind and have a "flesh-a-thon." Ever have one of those? It's kind of like a pity party, but with more food. Then I discovered the wisdom of having a plan B. If I did my best to follow God, eat within healthy guidelines, and get some physical activity in during the day, I knew I was still making progress toward my goal. I was simply choosing to follow plan B that day.

Having a plan B and even a plan C also helps guard against an attack of guilt that could lead to emotional eating and other setbacks. The enemy of your soul would like nothing more than for you to try to do everything perfectly—and fail miserably. So, "do not give the devil a foothold,"[10] and have a workable plan B!

When to Exercise:

Exercising before eating helps you to eat less and keep your metabolism up so you will burn calories more efficiently.

- 30 to 45 minutes *before* breakfast, lunch, or dinner
- 1½ hours *after* breakfast, lunch, or dinner
- 10- to 15-minute segments throughout the day
- 30 to 45 minutes *after* your mid-morning or mid-afternoon snack
- slump time—that period of time around 3:00 or 4:00 p.m. when your energy dips and your focus isn't as sharp. Get up and move around for a few minutes to get your blood pumping. Drink some water and eat your mid-afternoon healthy snack.
- Become an active person. Take the stairs, stretch when you stand up, park farther away from the store, incorporate strengthening and stretch moves while on the telephone, stand up straight, and start seeing yourself as a vibrant, elegant, and active individual.

Exercise as to the Lord

One of the secrets I've discovered to making exercise a daily habit is combining activity with a spiritual discipline I'm already doing on a regular basis, such as praying or speaking scriptural affirmations.

Whatever we do "as to the Lord" is more than physical exercise—it's an act of worship. This is the primary difference between *BASIC Steps* and other systems available. This is the "In Christ" component of "Body And Soul In Christ." For the Christian, exercise is no longer drudgery. It is a joy. And "the joy of the LORD is your strength."[11]

Whenever I have asked a woman if she would be willing to take ten minutes to pray for her family, she said she would gladly do so. "Now, combine that with a walk," I suggest. "Walk away from your house for five minutes while praying for your family. After five minutes, turn around and come back praising God for answering your prayers and blessing each family member." She will often exclaim, "Wow! I can do that!"

A Daily Walk with the Lord's Prayer

"And when you pray, do not use vain repetitions as the heathen do. For they think that they will be heard for their many words. Therefore do not be like them. For your Father knows the things you have need of before you ask Him. In this manner, therefore, pray: Our Father in heaven, hallowed be Your name."[12]

Most of us lead demanding lives. Obligations to family, work, and church leave us little time for ourselves. The loud clamor of life in the fast lane can squeeze out our quiet time with God. As for physical exercise, we've already discovered that it's not optional. It's necessary if we are to lead a healthy life.

What if you found a way to combine quality devotional time with the Lord while exercising your body?

My pet name for "A Daily Walk with the Lord's Prayer" is "Running the Prayer Track." Like a runner, I'm following a track. It's a ten-step track, following the outline of the Lord's Prayer, that has the added bonus of keeping *me* on track!

After a quick muscle-building Gimme Ten Workout, I grab my Prayer Track card (check the resources section for ordering information) and go for a brisk walk or run either on the treadmill or outdoors. This has become a meaningful time the Lord and I share.

The beauty of "A Daily Walk with the Lord's Prayer" is that you don't have to exercise to use it. My pastor's wife, Elizabeth, said she enjoyed wearing the prayer cards around her neck to pray while doing chores around the house. She said it also reminded her that we're to keep the Word of God close to our hearts.

Sometimes I prefer to follow the prayer sequence during my quiet devotional time while sitting or kneeling before the Lord. My friend Karen used the prayer cards during a lengthy car trip along the California coast. She said the time seemed to fly.

Pray these ten steps for yourself. Pause after each step and meditate on what you have just said. The steps are simply guidelines. Add your own words. You may find yourself lingering on one step longer than others to pray, meditate, or praise. You may pray through the steps quickly on some days, slowly on others. I believe that the Lord will reveal Himself to you in new ways as you meditate on His Word. Allow Him to guide your prayers, and make Him the focal point of all your praise and worship.

Our Father
You are my Father.

in heaven,
You are in heaven; I am on the earth.

hallowed be Your name.
You are…

El Shaddai—Almighty God (You are the all-sufficient one)

Elohim—the Lord (You are the creator)

Jehovah-jireh—the Lord our provider

Jehovah-M'Kaddesh—the Lord our sanctifier (You set me apart and purify me)

Jehovah-nissi—the Lord our banner (You are my victory)

Jehovah-rapha—the Lord who heals

Jehovah-rohi—the Lord who sees (You are my shepherd and guide)

Jehovah-shalom—the Lord our peace

Jehovah-shammah—the Lord who is present (You are always with me)

Jehovah-tsidekenu—the Lord our righteousness

Your kingdom come, Your will be done on earth as it is in heaven.

Father, I pray for the peace of Jerusalem.[13]

I declare Your will be done in our country. Bless our leaders and protect us.[14]

Let Your will be done in our church and its leaders.

May Your Word be proclaimed throughout the world.

I declare Your will is being done in my family.

Let Your will be done in my life. Show me Your vision for me, and lead me to fulfill Your goals for me.

Give us this day our daily bread.

Thank You for Your provision in every area of my life: spiritual, physical, emotional, social, and financial.[15]

Thank You for giving me favor with everyone I meet.[16]

I expect miracles today and every day!

I joyfully give you my tithe and offerings, and I give alms to the poor. I also joyfully receive![17]

And forgive us our debts,

I repent. I ask Your forgiveness, and I turn away from sinful ways.

Thank You for Your forgiveness, and I now receive Your cleansing from all unrighteousness.[18]

I owe no man anything but love.[19]

as we forgive our debtors.

Father, I forgive _____ and let go of all bitterness. I release this person to You and set myself free.

As You have forgiven me, I forgive myself and others.

I go on in strength, peace, and joy with You.

And do not lead us into temptation,

Father, I trust You to guide me by Your Word and wisdom.

By faith I apply the blood of Jesus to the doorposts of my life and the lives of my family members.[20]

I am strong in the Lord and the power of His might.

I put on the whole armor of God:

the belt of truth

the breastplate of righteousness

the preparation of the gospel of peace

the shield of faith

the helmet of salvation

the sword of the Spirit, which is the Word of God[21]

but deliver us from the evil one.

Thank You, Jesus, for defeating Satan and returning me to my right place in You.

Thank You for giving me victory in every area of my life.

The enemy is a liar, he has been defeated, and he's under my feet!

I have authority over the enemy, and no plan against my family will defeat us.

Thank You, Father, for giving Your angels charge over my family and me to keep us safe in all our ways.[22]

For Yours is the kingdom and the power and the glory forever. Amen.

Father, I praise You with my whole heart!

I love You! I thank You! I adore You!

Oh, how I delight in being Your child and knowing You as my loving Father!

I will now listen to You as You speak to my heart.[23]

Put Some Muscle in It

The quicker we get some more lean muscle working for you, the quicker you will reach your fitness goals. Muscle is a good thing—your heart's a muscle. And muscle burns fat (we like that!). One pound of muscle burns about 35 calories a day, but one pound of fat burns only two calories a day.

If we don't practice strength training, we begin to lose muscle, and the rate at which this occurs increases with age. As we lose muscle, our metabolism slows, we burn fewer calories, and we gain fat. For instance, say that between the ages of 35 and 45, a woman has lost ten pounds of muscle and gained about ten pounds of fat. That means she could get on the scale and weigh the same as she did ten years ago, but her dresses are two sizes larger than they were ten years ago. Why is that? Well, even though muscle weighs about four times more than fat, it takes up a lot less room than fat. Five pounds of fat takes up more than twice the space of five pounds of muscle. That's why a lean, athletic woman may weigh 130 pounds and wear a size 4 dress, while a nonathletic woman weighing 130 pounds might wear a size 10 dress. It's like the difference between five pounds of marshmallows and five pounds of gold.

By the way, weight training will *not* turn you into Mr. Universe, ladies! And don't make the mistake of thinking that if you do muscle training *before* you reach your ideal weight you'll become Miss Chunky-Muscle girl. No, the muscle will actually help you lose fat *faster*. More muscle increases your metabolic rate. If you increased your lean body mass by only five pounds (losing five pounds of fat and gaining five pounds of lean muscle), you would increase your metabolic rate by about 175 calories a day. Ten pounds of lean muscle would expend 350 more calories a day. Can you see with more muscle you don't have to concern yourself about calories as much? You're burnin' 'em up!

What if you're already slim and gorgeous? You need weight training too. Every woman does—and men too, of course. If you don't do resistance training, you will lose muscle as you age. That's why people who have always been slim wonder why they gain weight as they age. "I'm eating the same as I always have," they say. Losing muscle is the culprit. Less muscle means lower metabolism, fewer calories burned, and more fat.

Ten Minutes a Day

This will be the strength-training portion of your workout. You will still need to perform an aerobic activity three to five days a week. If you want to lose weight, I strongly recommend doing this *easy* ten-minute workout six days a week. That's just ten minutes out of every day—the same amount of time as it takes to drive up to a fast-food restaurant and get your order, or wait in line at the supermarket or bank. It's a ridiculously small price to pay for the tremendous benefits you'll receive in the form of increased muscle, a leaner body, and more energy and self-esteem (you will feel *so* good about yourself after each workout—I promise!).

If you don't want to lose weight, I'd still recommend doing the Gimme Ten Workout three to five days a week to enhance and maintain your muscular strength. All adults should do some form of strength training.

This is a great workout for beginners, so when you're ready to advance to something more difficult—go for it! I'd suggest seeing a certified personal trainer at a local gym who can design a plan for you and help you reach your goals.

You will need a set of dumbbells—three, five, or eight pounds each. Make sure they're light enough to feel comfortable but heavy enough to challenge you. A good way to test the weights is this: If you can do 12 repetitions of an exercise and feel your muscle fatigued (but not hurting), that's the right weight for you. If your muscle is *not* tired, try a heavier weight.

At any time if you feel pain, *stop!* My saying is "No pain, no pain. *Please* no pain."

You will be alternating between upper- and lower-body workouts. For fast results, I recommend doing Gimme Ten on Monday through Saturday and taking Sunday off. On Monday, Wednesday, and Friday, choose an aerobic activity to do after Gimme Ten. This could be a brisk 20 to 45 minute walk outdoors or on the treadmill following "A Daily Walk with the Lord's Prayer" or cycling, swimming, rebounding—whatever aerobic activity you choose. Alternate between different aerobic activities now and then so your body won't get used to the same routines all the time.

On Tuesday, Thursday, and Saturday, follow Gimme Ten with a PraiseMoves routine or other flexibility training. This way you're working your whole body and developing fitness in three ways: aerobics (for cardiovascular health, fat burning, and endurance), weight training (for lean body mass and strength), and stretches (for joint mobility, balance, and flexibility).

Guidelines

1. Do one minute of warm-ups while saying or meditating on the corresponding Scripture.
2. Do four strength moves for one minute each.
3. Repeat the four strength moves again for one minute each.
4. End with a one-minute stretch while meditating on a line of Scripture.

If you would rather have a visual aid to follow the workout, please check out the resources section to order the Gimme Ten Workout video or DVD and other products, including our spoken Scripture-to-Music collection (Scriptures set to upbeat praise music for workouts and walking, or beautiful praise hymns for stretches and relaxing). Please note that standing exercises may be done while sitting.

The Gimme Ten Workout

MONDAY

Upper-Body Workout

1. Warm-up: jog, march, or dance in place to music (one minute)

   Repeat this Scripture: *"I can do all things through Christ who strengthens me."*[24]

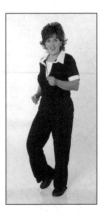

2. Bicep curls with weights (one minute)
   - Begin with arms at side, elbows straight, palms up, weights in hand
   - Bend elbows upward
   - Return to starting position
   - Repeat

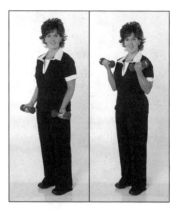

3. Triceps kickbacks with weights (one minute)
   - Straighten elbow back
   - Return to starting position

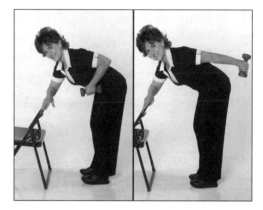

4. Shoulder overhead press with weights (can be done one arm at a time) (one minute)
   - Elbows bent, hold weights in hands at shoulders
   - Lift weights up and overhead
   - Return to starting position and repeat

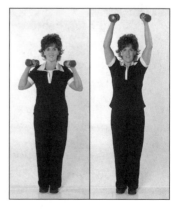

5. Push-ups on bent knees (or standing, push against a wall) (one minute)

- Lie facedown on floor, hands by shoulders
- Bend knees, cross ankles
- Push up, keeping knees bent, straighten elbows, back straight
- Lower and repeat

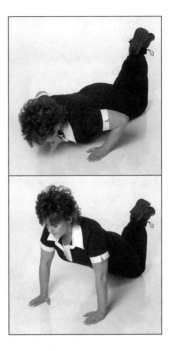

6. Repeat exercises 2 through 5

7. Stretching and relaxation (one minute)

- Sit on floor, right leg out, left foot against right thigh
- Gently bend over, resting hands where comfortable
- Relax neck
- Repeat on other side

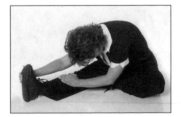

Meditate on this Scripture: *"He is my glory and the One who lifts up my head."* [25]

Add 20 to 45 minutes of brisk walking for aerobic exercise.

Lower-Body Workout

1. Warm-up: jog, march, or dance in place to music (one minute)

   Repeat this Scripture: *"The LORD is my shepherd; I shall not want."*[26]

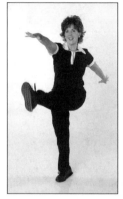

2. Calf raises (one minute)
   - Stand, using chair for balance
   - Rise up on toes, tightening calves
   - Repeat

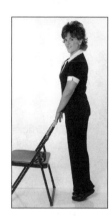

3. Forward lunge with weights (one minute)
   - Stand, holding weights
   - Step forward, keeping torso straight
   - Push back to starting position

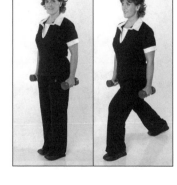

4. Crunches with arms folded (one minute)

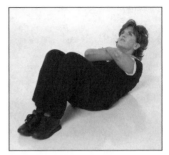

- Lie on back, knees bent, arms across chest
- Slowly curl up, lifting head and shoulders
- Look at ceiling, pull stomach in
- Keep lower back touching floor
- Slowly lower back to starting position
- Repeat

5. Lower tummy tuck with leg raises (one minute)

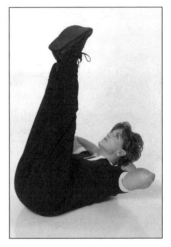

- Lie on back, hands behind head
- Lift legs, toes pointing up
- Gently lift head, looking at ceiling
- Lift hips, feeling pull in lower abdomen—this is a very small movement
- Lift and lower hips in small, gentle movements—no rocking

6. Repeat exercises 2 through 5

7. Stretching and relaxation (one minute)

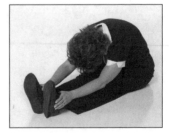

- Both legs straight
- Keep knees soft
- Gently fold over legs and hold wherever comfortable
- Relax completely

Meditate on this Scripture: *"With God all things are possible."*[27]

Add 20 to 45 minutes of PraiseMoves for flexibility and stress relief.

Upper-Body Workout

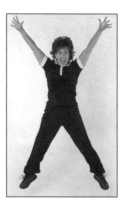

1. Warm-up: jog, march, or dance in place to music (one minute)

   Repeat this Scripture: *"Jesus Christ is the same yesterday, today, and forever."*[28]

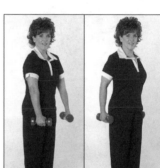

2. Shoulder rolls with weights (one minute)
   - Raise shoulders upward toward ears and roll them backward
   - Roll shoulders forward to starting position
   - Repeat

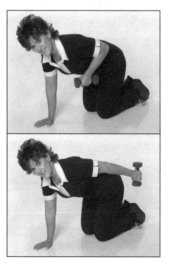

3. Kneeling tricep kickbacks (or Monday's standing tricep kickbacks) (one minute)
   - Start on hands and knees, elbow bent, weight in right hand
   - Straighten elbow back
   - Return to starting position
   - Repeat several times and then repeat on the left side

4. Push-ups on bent knees (or standing, push against a wall) (one minute)
   - Lie on floor, facedown, hands by shoulders
   - Bend knees, cross ankles
   - Push up, keeping knees bent, straighten elbows, back straight
   - Lower and repeat

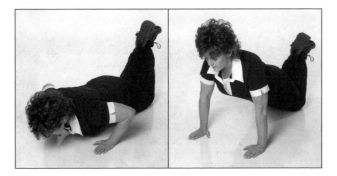

5. Standing row with weights (one minute)
   - Stand, arms straight in front, weights touching
   - Lift weights up, elbows at shoulder level
   - Lower and repeat

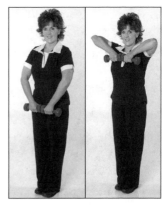

6. Repeat exercises 2 through 5

7. Stretching and relaxation (alternate legs) (one minute)

   Meditate on this Scripture: *"Wisdom is the principal thing."*[29]

   Add 20 to 45 minutes of brisk walking for aerobic exercise.

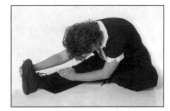

Lower-Body Workout

1. Warm-up: jog, march, or dance in place to music (one minute)

   Repeat this Scripture: *"The Lord is my light and my salvation."*[30]

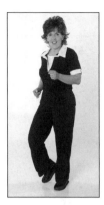

2. One-legged calf raise (one minute)
   - Stand, using chair for balance
   - Rise up onto ball of right foot, lower slowly, repeat several times
   - Repeat with left foot

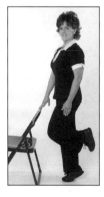

3. Lunge squats with weights (one minute)
   - Hold weights in hands
   - Step right foot forward, keeping torso straight
   - Bend knees bringing torso straight down, not forward
   - Do not let the front knee go beyond the toes
   - Repeat several times
   - Switch to the left leg

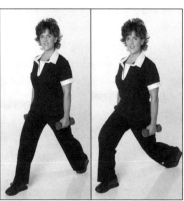

4. Diagonal crunches (one minute)
   - Lie on back, knees bent, hands behind head
   - Lift head, reaching right arm across body toward the left, pulling in abdominal muscles
   - Do not pull neck
   - Gently pulse
   - Lower and repeat on the other side

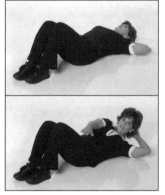

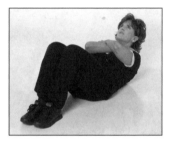

5. Crunches with arms folded (one minute)
   - Lie on back, knees bent, arms across chest
   - Slowly curl up, lifting head and shoulders
   - Look at ceiling, pull stomach in
   - Keep lower back touching floor
   - Slowly lower back to starting position
   - Repeat

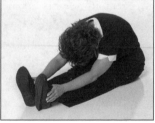

6. Repeat exercises 2 through 5

7. Stretching and relaxation (one minute)

   Meditate on this Scripture: *"God has not given us a spirit of fear, but of power and of love and of a sound mind."*[31]

   Add 20 to 45 minutes of Praise-Moves for flexibility and stress relief.

Upper-Body Workout

1. Warm-up: jog, march, or dance in place to
   music (one minute)

   Repeat this Scripture: *"I have come that they
   may have life, and that they may have it more
   abundantly."*[32]

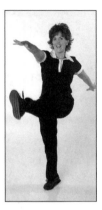

2. Triceps kickbacks with weights (one minute)
   - Stand, leaning over chair, arm back, elbow bent, weight in
     hand
   - Straighten elbow back
   - Return to starting position

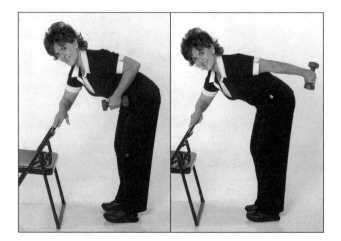

3. Push-ups on bent knees (or standing, push against a wall) (one minute)
   - Lie facedown on floor, hands by shoulders
   - Bend knees, cross ankles
   - Push up, keeping knees bent, straighten elbows, back straight
   - Lower and repeat

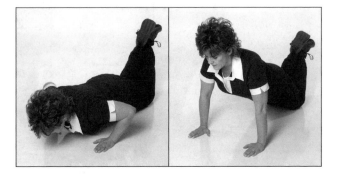

4. Alternating bicep curls with weights (one minute)
   - Begin with arms at side, elbows straight, palms up, weights in hand
   - Bend right elbow upward
   - Return to starting position
   - Repeat on left side, alternating bicep curls slowly and evenly

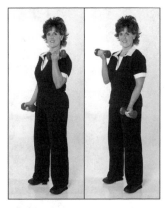

5. Standing row with weights (one minute)
   - Stand, arms straight down in front, weights touching
   - Lift weights up, elbows at shoulder level
   - Lower and repeat

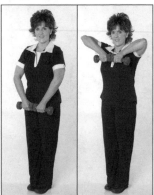

6. Repeat exercises 2 through 5

7. Stretching and relaxation
   (alternate legs) (one minute)

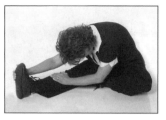

Meditate on this Scripture: *"Christ has redeemed us from the curse of the law."*[33]

Add 20 to 45 minutes of brisk walking for aerobic exercise.

Lower-Body Workout

1. Warm-up: jog, march, or dance in place
   to music (one minute)

   Repeat this Scripture: *"And my God shall supply all your need according to His riches in glory by Christ Jesus."*[34]

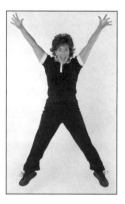

2. Knee squats with weights (one
   minute)
   • Stand straight, weights in
     hands
   • Bend knees to 90 degrees
   • Straighten knees
   • Repeat

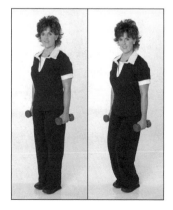

3. Inner thigh raise (one minute)
   - Lie on side, resting on elbow, top leg bent with foot on floor
   - Lift bottom leg, using your inner thigh and hip muscles
   - Hold, lower, repeat
   - After several raises, switch to other side

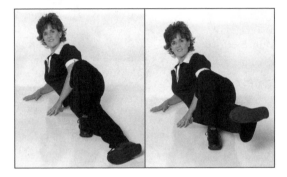

4. Outer thigh raise (one minute)
   - Lie on side, resting on elbow
   - Raise top leg as high as possible using outer thigh and hip muscles
   - Hold, lower, repeat
   - After several raises, switch sides

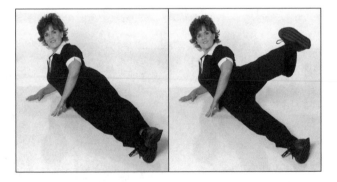

5. Abdomen and lumbar knee raises (one minute)
- Lie on back with knees bent and feet flat on floor
- Don't arch back
- Lift hips off floor
- Raise and straighten right leg, hold, and return foot to floor
- Repeat with left leg
- Continue to alternate raising legs, keeping hips off the floor

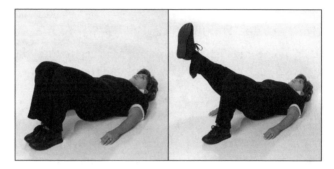

6. Repeat exercises 2 through 5

7. Stretching and relaxation (one minute)

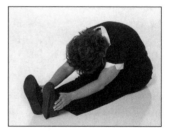

Meditate on this Scripture: *"Give, and it will be given to you: good measure, pressed down, shaken together, and running over."*[35]

Add 20 to 45 minutes of PraiseMoves for flexibility and stress relief.

Activity Throughout the Day

How can you incorporate activity and strength-building exercises into your day? You can do isometrics while sitting at the computer or watching television. Isometrics are exercises that tense muscles briefly (such as placing the palms of your hands together in front of your chest and pressing for a count of eight to work the muscles of the arms and chest). While on the telephone, use hand-held weights to work your biceps, and do calf stretches, leg lifts, and gentle knee bends.

A Journey of 10,000 Steps Begins with One...

...pedometer! A simple pedometer can keep track of the miles you walk as you go about your day. Walking 10,000 steps a day equals about five miles and burns as many calories as 30 minutes of exercise. You can burn 2000 to 3500 extra calories a week this way—and what happens when you burn 3500 calories? Right! One pound of fat is gone!

Two thousand steps equals about one mile. Challenge yourself and increase your steps over a four-week period, building up to 10,000 or more per day. Sitting at a computer all day makes that difficult, so schedule times to get up and move.

Wearing a pedometer during the day will be an eye-opener for some who think all they do is walk all day (perhaps they don't). Those who think they don't do much by chasing kids around the house may be surprised to see how many steps they do take throughout the day. Continuous aerobic activity for at least 20 minutes is important for cardiovascular health and is different from the start-and-stop walking around we do during the day. Four thousand steps (two miles) walked continuously over a 30-minute period has more aerobic benefit than 4000 steps walked over a 16-hour period.

On the Rebound

You can do a great workout on the rebounder, or mini-trampoline. It exercises all parts of the body at once and is very easy on the joints. Rebounding stimulates the lymphatic system, so it also acts as a detoxifier. People of any age can use a rebounder—and it's fun! Those who are ill or unable to jump on the rebounder can benefit from sitting on the rebounder while someone else bounces gently on it.

Rebounders vary in quality and usually cost between $20 and $200.

Quick Tips

Don't like to exercise alone? Exercise with a friend—someone who will keep you accountable!

Set goals and reward yourself as you attain them. This can be something small, such as "I'll watch my favorite TV show *after* I do my Gimme Ten workout." When you reach a bigger goal, reward yourself in other ways (buying a book or a piece of clothing you've wanted, going to lunch with a friend, or relaxing in a hot bath with lots of bubbles).

Aim high but be realistic. It's better to say, "I'm going to walk 20 minutes a day five days a week" than "I'm going to walk more." Be specific.

Chart your progress, but don't be addicted to the scale. Throw it away (or put it in the closet). Since you're going to be gaining lean muscle (which weighs more than fat), you might get discouraged to see you've gained a pound. You may actually have lost fat and been gaining lean muscle, so the scale is not an accurate judge of the state of your fitness. Chart your progress in other ways, such as in keeping a journal of your progress, prayers, emotional growth, and new ideas.

Mix it up! Change your routine around every so often. Challenge yourself, walk a different route, take a ballet class, exercise with your children...do something different.

Bringing It Home

In this chapter I learned...

1. _____

2. _____

3. _____

I can start doing this better today: _____

_____

Lord, I ask You to help me _____

_____

Step Two

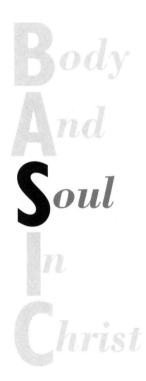

Body
And
Soul
In
Christ

5

Renewing Your Mind:
Where Godly Fitness Begins

And do not be conformed to this world,
but be transformed by the renewing of your mind,
that you may prove what is that good and
acceptable and perfect will of God.

ROMANS 12:2

You ARE A *SPIRIT* WHO HAS A *SOUL,* and you live in a *body.* Your soul consists of your mind, will, and emotions. What's on *your* mind? Researchers estimate that we think about 60,000 thoughts per day at a speed of 600 to 800 words per minute. Do you find your thoughts consistently running along positive paths or negative ones? When something bad happens, do you think, *It figures. Nothing good ever happens to me.* Or do you think, *I'm not moved by this. God said, "Many are the afflictions of the righteous, but the* LORD *delivers him out of them all."*[1] *I'm coming out of this one too.*

Quoting Scripture may be new to you, but it's certainly better than quoting many of the slogans the world hands us. "If it feels good, do it" has landed people in more jams than Smuckers. How about the woeful outlook of Murphy's Law, which says if anything can go wrong, it probably will?

We're made in the image of God, and we're told to imitate Him as His dear children.[2] One way we do that is by thinking and speaking His words.

Faith Comes by Hearing, and Hearing…

What do imitators of God say, and how do they say it? Believers use their faith to say aloud and believe the promises of God found in the Bible. The more you say the Word of God and hear it coming out of your own mouth, the more your faith will grow.[3] Since faith is not mere wishing, but the "substance of things hoped for,"[4] your breakthrough is based on your faith. Faith is the substance out of which your fondest hopes and desires are made. In Greek, the word for "substance" is *hupóstasis,* which means "foundation, existence, or confident expectation."[5]

I heard a Bible teacher call faith your "title deed." I like that. When you have a title deed to a property, you know it's yours. The property may be in another state, but as long as you have that title in your name, the property is yours. The promises in the Bible are yours as well. Because you're a child of God, they've got your name on them. You can claim them just as you would a property or inheritance legally granted to you.

Here's a practical example of how you can use the Word of God to overcome an everyday challenge. Let's say you've made the commitment to take better care of the marvelous temple the Lord's given you, so you determine to follow "A Daily Walk with the Lord's Prayer" first thing in the morning. Your body tells your mind, I'm *too tired to take a walk today. I don't feel like it.* Your mind says, *Well, it* is *cloudy outside. It's probably not a good idea. Let's go later.* Remember that you are first and foremost a spirit made in the image of God. You have a soul consisting of your mind, will, and emotions, and you live in an "earth suit"—your body. If you allow your carnal nature to dominate, your spirit will remain weak. However, you can make the decision that you will not be controlled by thoughts and feelings. Instead, overrule your flesh with Philippians 4:13: "I can do all things through Christ who strengthens me."

Feelings have nothing to do with faith. Faith operates on a higher level than feelings. In fact, whenever I follow my feelings instead of faith, I wind up off track and miserable. My body rarely wants to do what my spirit wants to do. It has to be trained.

So you decide to live by the Spirit as you care for your body. You choose to not blend into the couch today—or tomorrow. You cultivate the fruit of self-control by getting up, putting one foot in front of the other, and walking. Your mind is being transformed by the Word of God.

The apostle Paul wrote, "I discipline my body like an athlete, training it to do what it should. Otherwise, I fear that after preaching to others I myself might be disqualified."[6] The King James Version says, "I myself should be a castaway." A castaway! That refers to someone who is shipwrecked and discarded. If we cannot discipline ourselves physically, we will more and more easily say no to God in other areas of life as well. What if God has a great work for us to do that will require discipline and physical stamina to fulfill? If we give in to every whim of the flesh, can God trust us with more significant tasks?

For years it felt like I was treading water spiritually. The desires of the Lord were in my heart, but I lacked the discipline to see them through. I was disobedient and undisciplined, especially in the areas of food and exercise. Like an unruly child, my flesh did not respond well to the word *no*. I felt like I was at war with my body, mind, and emotions. One of the most powerful tools I've found to train the flesh is fasting, which we'll look at in chapter 8. I didn't want my habits and carnal desires to stand in the way of the plans and purposes God has for my life. Since "he who is faithful in what is least is faithful also in much,"[7] I realized that being unfaithful in little can just as easily lead to being unfaithful in much.

Having no dietary restraints can lead to unrestrained behavior in other areas as well. Lasciviousness and lust do not limit themselves to sexual perversion. The greedy, grasping, and selfish desire to keep the best piece of food for myself goes counter to the law of love, which tells us to give. The flesh screams, *I gotta have it now!* while our spirit says, *Let's yield to the spiritual fruit of patience and self-control.*

We are to walk in love, live by faith, and speak faith-filled words. When we meditate upon and speak God's Word, we are not just saying positive, pie-in-the-sky affirmations; we are speaking in agreement with what God says about us!

Some may ask, "But am I being hypocritical if I'm quoting Scriptures that are different from what I'm experiencing?" Let's ask Abraham and Sarah. God began speaking His desired result into their lives long before they saw a change in their natural situation. They were childless, and Sarah was physically incapable of having a child. When Abram was 75 years old, God changed his name to Abraham, which means "father of many nations." This was 25 years before Abraham fathered Isaac—when he was 100 years old!

Hebrew names in Bible days had greater meaning than our names today. Abraham consistently heard the promise of God whenever he introduced himself. "Hello, I am the father of many nations," he would say. His name helped keep his faith strong until the promise of God was fulfilled in his life and Isaac was born. Interestingly, Isaac means "laughter." You know people must have laughed and praised the Lord with Sarah and Abraham when a formerly barren 90-year-old woman and 100-year-old man had their first child! God is faithful.

Think About It

Have you ever had a horrible thought come to mind? We all have. You may have heard people say, "Thoughts are like birds. You can't stop the birds from flying over your head, but you can sure stop them from building a nest in your hair!" Ever wonder where those terrible thoughts originate? We know that only good things come from God,[8] so these other thoughts come from either our own mind or Satan.

As a teenager I read horror novels and watched scary movies to frighten myself out of my wits. I think it worked, because I did some pretty witless stunts in my misspent youth. Some of those images came back to me from time to time. Our minds store images we've seen over the years. Now, by the grace of God and the sacrifice made by the shed blood of Jesus Christ, we can be cleansed from the sins of the past and the images that trouble us. Ask Him to forgive you for allowing yourself to be drawn into unwholesome entertainment and habits (this includes pornography, violence, foul language, and other ungodly pursuits that feed the lust of the flesh). Include with this all of your negative thoughts about yourself—you know, the *I'm a fat, ugly, stupid, good-for-nothing, useless nerd* thoughts that were planted in your mind over the years. Ask the Lord to cleanse you from all unrighteousness[9] and purge those images and thoughts from your mind.

A friend of mine I'll call Carol is a young mother. She confided in me that horrible images kept coming to her mind whenever she was driving. She would see herself involved in a terrible accident. The images caused her to worry throughout the day, and she was becoming an increasingly nervous driver. Her thoughts affected her judgment. I saw this as a weapon from the enemy sent against her to fulfill the plan of Satan against her life. We prayed and bound the enemy according to Matthew 18:18. We thanked God for His protection and His promise that "no weapon formed against you shall prosper."[10]

I shared some Scriptures with her that she could use to combat those thoughts and images if the enemy tried to use them against her again. Keeping away from violent images on television and in movies is also a wise decision. I have found most R-rated and PG-13 rated material opposes Christ-centered spiritual fitness. Months after our conversation, Carol told me those dreadful images never came back.

Carol's experience notwithstanding, don't be surprised if the enemy offers you a suggestion to meditate on thoughts and images from the past again. It's like erasing something from your computer. An on-screen message will pop up: "Are you sure you want to delete this?" These thoughts may have become such a part of you that you feel uncomfortable or strange meditating on good thoughts instead. The negative thoughts may try to come back, but remember those "birds" flying over your head—you don't have to let them build a nest in your hair.

Here's a recipe to keep in mind—literally! It's from Paul's letter to the church at Philippi:

> *Finally brethren, whatever things are true, whatever things are noble, whatever things are just, whatever things are pure, whatever things are lovely, whatever things are of good report, if there is any virtue and if there is anything praiseworthy—meditate on these things.*[11]

There's a Mouse in the House!

What can you do when a negative thought or image comes to mind? Don't meditate on it or worry about it. Capture it! What would you do if you found a mouse in the house—invite it to dinner? No! You'd capture and kill it (or at least send it over to the next county). Thoughts that don't line up with the Word of God deserve the same treatment. Let's say an old thought floats up from the past like a personal invitation to a one-woman pity party: *Nobody loves me.* If we meditate on that thought long enough, we'll wind up with our heads in the refrigerator weeping into the corn chips. On the other hand, we can capture that thought.

"For the weapons of our warfare are not physical [weapons of flesh and blood], but they are mighty before God for the overthrow and destructions of strongholds."[12]

A stronghold can be a fortress of protection or a prison. The Lord is our strong tower and fortress. In Him we have safety and peace. We might use addictions, habits, and patterns of thinking to escape from the pains of reality, but each action or thought can become a prison wall. Turning to food to relieve the emotional pain I felt as a child numbed me for a while, but the consequences were painful and long-lasting. Compulsive overeating trapped me in a prison.

The next verse says we are to "lead every thought and purpose away captive into the obedience of Christ."

Okay, so here's the moment of truth: *Nobody loves me.* The old thought flies in low under the radar, but you catch it. You've been renewing your mind on the Word of God, so that thought doesn't stand a chance. You immediately recognize it doesn't agree with Scripture, so you decide to arrest that thought before it can do any more damage. "I resist that thought in the name of Jesus," you say. Then you replace it with the truth. "The Word of God says I'm accepted in the Beloved."[13] Good job! Another prison wall bites the dust.

Here's one we all hear whining at us from time to time: *I can't do it. It's too hard.* My all-time favorite rebuttal for that one is "I can do all things through Christ who strengthens me."[14]

Each time we decide to cast down those imaginations and thoughts that are contrary to the Bible and choose to replace them with the Word of God, we are leading "every thought and purpose away captive into the obedience of Christ." We are tearing down the prison walls of the past and building up the fortress of the Lord. Soon those old thoughts will just bounce off that impenetrable tower. Haven't you found that some of the things that used to tempt you years ago don't hold the power over you they once did?

When I was a teenager, I got a sick thrill out of stealing things at department stores. I'd palm a lipstick or a package of panty hose and feel an addictive rush of adrenaline. My desperado career was shortened, thank God, when I was apprehended by a store detective.

Now that I have surrendered my life to Jesus Christ and have been renewing my mind through the Word, the reasons I don't steal have more to do with my desire to do right than with a desire not to get caught doing something wrong. If I suddenly thought, *Hey, why don't I just stick that eyeliner in my purse?* I would probably break out laughing. Stealing is no longer a temptation to me. The old prison has been torn down, and a new fortress stands in its place.

Take a look at the prisons that still stand in your life. They are built one brick at a time by your thoughts and actions. One blast from the Word of God, however, can start the process of tearing down those walls.

You Will Have Whatever You Say[15]

Why should you speak aloud what God says about you and your family, resisting any thoughts that are contrary to the Word of God? What you think about determines what you will say. What you say determines the choices and actions you will take. You will eventually experience what you continually think about and say. For example, the thought to raise your right arm comes before actually raising your right arm. Thought precedes action.

Proverbs 18:21 says, "Death and life are in the power of the tongue, and those who love it will eat its fruit." I think death was mentioned first for a reason. Our words can choke the life of the Spirit right out of us. We all know people who love to talk and seem to say whatever comes into their head without thinking first. I'll admit I've been guilty of that. I learned to ask the Holy Spirit to keep a close watch on my mouth and not let foolish or harmful words come out. Whenever a thought occurs to me that is not pure, lovely, or of good report[16] I have a choice to say it out loud, to meditate on it, or to cast it down. Just before opening my mouth, I'll sense a gentle nudge on the inside. Some call it a "check in the spirit." I've learned from experience to stop and not blurt out whatever was flying through my head just then. Rather, I'll ask in my heart, *What is it, Lord?* I will often sense His gentle guidance: *Don't say that.*

Here is the point of decision. God always gives us a choice. "If death and life are in the power of the tongue," which do we want? Do we want life with a little bit of death on the side? Of course not. Choose life, even if it seems to be the more difficult choice.

Choose life-affirming and pure entertainment, reading material, music, and friendships. Renew your mind through the Word of God by reading the Bible, attending Bible studies at church, speaking scriptural promises aloud, and listening to trusted Bible teachers. We control our thought life by filling our minds with good things. The thoughts we think guide the words we say, our decisions, and the actions we take. Our actions set the course of our lives. Are we filling our heads with *Days of Our Lives*, or are we setting our minds on heavenly things?[17]

The Bible gives us the perfect prescription: "Don't copy the behavior and customs of this world, but let God transform you into a new person by changing the way you think. Then you will know what God wants you to do, and you will know how good and pleasing and perfect His will really is."[18]

We are to *let* God transform us. We are a part of this process. Meditate on the Word of God and let it change the way you think. How do you meditate? If you know how to worry, you know how to meditate. Worry is meditating on what the devil wants to see happen in your life. I decided to give up worry when I realized that "whatever is not from faith is sin."[19] Similarly, when you contemplate a sentence or two of the Word of God over and over again in your mind, considering every angle, you are meditating. Next, ask the Holy Spirit to shine new light on the Scripture for you. Then speak the Word aloud so you can hear it for yourself; it will build your faith. This is the best prescription for life you'll find![20]

Self-Control: The Boundaries of Freedom

I realized I wasn't going to experience victory over the flesh without developing the fruit of self-control. Imposing restraints and boundaries on ourselves is something children and most adults don't like to do. It doesn't come naturally to us.

For me, developing self-control involved four things:

1. filling myself with the Word of God at every opportunity,

2. taming my tongue to speak according to the Word,

3. being honest about what I should and should not be eating, watching, reading, and doing, and then asking God to help me with the commitments I knew I had to make, and

4. sowing seeds of discipline.

Realizing that sugar and caffeine had adverse effects on me, I decided to stop eating foods containing them, as well as most processed foods. I played with the decision for months, but then I realized I had to make a commitment to God and myself that I was going to change—and mean it. Fasting for a few days was enormously helpful in ridding my body of the physical addiction to these substances, and it also cleared my mind to focus on God's will for my life.

A daily fellowship time with the Lord is also vital for spiritual growth, emotional balance, and victory over the flesh. The Step-UP program in chapter 10 will give you a good format to follow. I have found when I commit time to the Lord first thing in the morning, not only does my day go more smoothly, but I have time to do everything I need to do with the peace, wisdom, and knowledge of God to do it. When I used to "hit the ground runnin'," I never seemed to have enough time and was always having to clean up after the messes I made along the way. Knowing God's will (His Word) and having His wisdom can make all the difference between enjoying a good day or enduring a frenzied one.

Overcoming Temptations

Realize that temptations will come, just as they came to Jesus. Remember that He battled Satan with the Word of God and won. So can you.

Have you noticed that the enemy used food to tempt Adam and Eve in the garden and Jesus in the wilderness? Our diet certainly is a major area of attack for many of us. Satan offered Jesus the temptation of physical food after He had been fasting for 40 days. Immediately Jesus opposed him with the Word: "It is written, 'Man shall not live by bread alone, but by every word that proceeds from the mouth of God.'"[21]

Your victory over the flesh will not come from the perfect diet but from renewing your mind on the perfect Word of God and cultivating the fruits of self-control, faithfulness, and patience. When your mind is renewed through the Word, you will find yourself making choices that agree with the Word. Self-control will become easier. Decisions based on love will begin to win over decisions based on selfishness. The restraints you place on your life will no longer be grievous, but safe boundaries that bring you freedom and peace.

God will not allow you to be tempted beyond what you are able to tolerate or endure. "No temptation has overtaken you except such as is common to man; but God is faithful, who will not allow you to be tempted beyond what you are able, but with the temptation will also make the way of escape, that you may be able to bear it."[22] That refers to more than the temptation to overeat or not exercise. It includes the temptation to give up standing in faith. If you are trusting in God's Word, believing He will fulfill His promises, you will often be tempted to quit. You can escape that temptation through prayer, speaking the Word aloud, thanking God for giving you victory, singing praises—whatever will stir your faith to *believe* the truth in spite of the temporary circumstances screaming the opposite message at you.

Faith is a noun, but *believe* is a verb, an action. One definition of *believe* that has helped me understand it better is this: "take *action* on the Word of God." That makes sense, doesn't it? Since "faith without works is dead,"[23] believing is *acting* on the Word regardless of what the circumstances may say. Circumstances are temporary and subject to change. Truth, however, is eternal. The Word of God is truth.

Paul tells us, "We do not look at the things which are seen, but at the things which are not seen. For the things which are seen are temporary, but the things which are not seen are eternal."[24] Since God has already given us "all things that pertain to life and godliness,"[25] we have the answer to our prayers by faith in Him.

God Knows What You Are Able to Bear

If you could not be victorious in this difficult situation you're facing, God would never have allowed you to experience it in the first place. Regardless of how seemingly insurmountable the odds may seem against you, God has a way out. He hasn't brought you this far to drop you now, and He certainly isn't going to let you make Him look bad because you stood in faith. He says we will never be ashamed when we trust in Him.[26]

God knew I could never come out of alcoholism myself, so the moment I surrendered my life to Jesus Christ, He immediately delivered me, and I never desired another drink. Giving up smoking was different—it took some faith, but He helped me. I've been free of that addiction now for many years, thank God. Being healed of compulsive overeating has been a process for me, one in which I must remain vigilant to *remain* free. I'm reminded of the ten lepers who were healed by Jesus "as they went."[27] Just keep walking, believing, and receiving.

God knew I could bear the temptations and overcome smoking and overeating, but not alcohol. In His infinite wisdom, He had mercy on me that day when I came to the end of myself.

On April Fool's Day, 1987, I went from being a fool for the world to a "fool for Christ." I cried out to God and said, "I surrender! I give up! You win." I was lonely and alone. God will use whatever it takes to bring you to your knees. For me it was loneliness. I wanted to get married. I wanted someone in my life who would love me for myself. "I've made a mess of my life," I said. "You're welcome to it if You can do something with it."

Desperately wanting love in my life, I cried, "If You want me to be alone, give me peace. If you want me to be with someone, then send him soon, because I can't live like this anymore." I fell onto my knees and then onto my face, and I felt a weight I'd always thought was part of the physical weight of my body lift off me. I later learned this was the weight of sin. Peace descended upon me for the first time in my life, and I cried happy tears. Four days later I met Paul, and we were married three months later on the Fourth of July (what we call "Interdependence Day!"). God answers prayer!

Present Your Body

The apostle Paul pleads with us in Romans 12:1 to present our bodies as living sacrifices to God, calling this our reasonable, rational service. I too urge you to present your body to God. Present your mind and what you meditate upon. Present your eyes and ears and what you allow into these gateways to the soul. Present your tongue and the words you say. Ask the Lord to keep watch over your mouth. Present your body as a living sacrifice and offer sacrifices of praise to Him with your whole heart. If you will do this, I promise you will indeed prove to yourself "what is that good and acceptable and perfect will of God."[28]

Terrific Tongue Tamers

These are examples of scriptural affirmations (not direct quotes but first-person declarations based on Scripture). Meditate on them, speak them aloud, and let their truths renew your mind.

- I am strong in the Lord and the power of His might (Ephesians 6:10).

- I can do all things through Christ who strengthens me (Philippians 4:13).

- The joy of the Lord is my strength (Nehemiah 8:10).

- The Lord is the strength of my life (Psalm 27:1).

- My body is a temple of the Holy Spirit (1 Corinthians 6:19).

- I present my body a living sacrifice, holy and acceptable to God, which is my reasonable service (Romans 12:1).

- (Act this next one out!) I put on the whole armor of God that I may be able to stand in the evil day. My waist is girded about with truth. I've put on the breastplate of righteousness. My feet are shod with the preparation of the gospel of peace. Above all, I take the shield of faith and quench all the fiery darts of the enemy. I take the helmet of salvation and the sword of the Spirit, which is the Word of God (Ephesians 6:13-17).

- The Word of God is a lamp to my feet and a light to my path (Psalm 119:105).

- Wisdom is the principal thing; therefore, I will get wisdom. And with all my getting, I will get understanding (Proverbs 4:7).

- I give attention to God's words and listen to His sayings. I keep them before my eyes and in my heart, for they are life and health to me. I keep my heart with all diligence, for out of it flow the issues of life. I choose not to have a deceitful mouth or perverse lips (Proverbs 4:20-24).

- Greater is He who is in me than he who is in the world (1 John 4:4).

- I discipline my body and bring it into subjection so that when I have preached to others, I will not become disqualified (1 Corinthians 9:27).
- I delight myself in the Lord, and He gives me the desires of my heart (Psalm 37:4).

Bringing It Home

In this chapter, I learned...

1. _____

2. _____

3. _____

I can start doing this better today: _____

_____

Lord, I ask You to help me _____

_____

6

Emotions: Forgiveness, the Key to Answered Prayer

*And whenever you stand praying, if you have
anything against anyone, forgive him, that your Father
in heaven may also forgive you your trespasses.
But if you do not forgive, neither will our Father
in heaven forgive your trespasses.*

MARK 11:25-26

FORGIVENESS IS AN ACT OF YOUR WILL. Like everything God commands us to do, it is for our benefit, and we are to do it in faith, regardless of our feelings. Forgiveness and unforgiveness effect our emotions, but they are not emotions. We choose to forgive because God wants us to, just as we choose to walk in unconditional love regardless of how we feel.

Forgiveness is not a sign of weakness, nor is it saying you're a doormat or suddenly accepting unacceptable behavior. It doesn't excuse a person from judgment; instead, it takes judgment from your hands and puts it in the hands of God, where it belongs.

Unforgiveness is poison to the spirit, soul, and body. We may think we are torturing the ones who hurt us by keeping them locked up in our mental prison, yet we are the ones held captive. Bitterness, anger, resentment—are all rooted in unforgiveness.

When I belonged to a 12-step program for compulsive overeaters, I learned that forgiveness was going to be a major part of my recovery.

I heard one person say, "A lot of that fat you're dealing with is unforgiveness and unexpressed anger." That seemed a little far-fetched to me until I remembered all the times I felt anger toward someone, and instead of expressing my emotions, I ate. In my old life, I would "drink at" the person or situation that angered or frustrated me. As a new Christian, I no longer drank alcohol or smoked cigarettes, so I returned to my original drug of choice—food—and my body showed it.

How about you? When you think of that one person (or group of persons) who hurt you, do you feel a sinking feeling or knot in the pit of your stomach? Perhaps your face flushes with anger, and your jaw clenches just thinking of them. If so, you know in your heart you have not released them into the Lord's hands, which is an apt description of forgiveness.

Unforgiveness is at the root of many unanswered prayers. It is like an impenetrable shield of brass between us and God. Refusing to let go of the wrongs done to us keeps prayers from being answered[1] and may be at the root of many physical illnesses as well.[2] It affects relationships with your spouse, your children, and others.

Make a List

If you are serious about walking in peace and victory, I cannot overemphasize the importance of forgiveness. You may have noticed I like to keep things simple. Making a list of people to forgive is the simplest way I know to release yourself from bondage to the past.

When you think briefly of your childhood, does anyone spring to mind whom you need to forgive? Write down that person's name. What about your teenage years? Don't go looking for something that's not there, but write down the name of anyone who immediately comes to mind. How about your young adult years? Your years as an adult? Your past few months?

Now write down what each person did that you need to forgive him or her for. Don't take too long—this is just a way for you to sort out your thoughts. It's important to separate the sin from the sinner when forgiving others. People are not our enemy—Satan is.

Please join with me in prayer.

Dear heavenly Father, I do not want to be held in bondage to the pain of the past. Please bring to my remembrance everyone I need to forgive so I can release them to You. I

want nothing to stand between You and me. Thank You for
guiding me through this process in obedience to Your Word.

Now go through the list and offer a simple prayer from your heart
to God. When I first did this, I said something like this out loud:
"Lord, I forgive John Smith. I release him into Your hands. I forgive him by faith in obedience to Your Word. From this point on I
know I have forgiven him and I am free from the pain, bitterness, and
resentment of the past in Jesus' name."

Forgiving Those No Longer Living

When I wrote my forgiveness list 15 years ago, a number of the
people I needed to release from my mental prison had already passed
away. Some of the wounds were old and deep. Several of these hurts
shaped the way I saw myself, affecting my confidence and ability to
trust others.

Forgiving my parents, who died in the early 1980s, was central to
my emotional healing. As I mentioned in the introduction, my
mother and I were very close. When she suffered mental and emotional illnesses during my childhood, our roles reversed, and I cared
for her even though I was a child myself.

I believe my mother knew and loved the Lord in her heart, but she
did not know how to live a victorious Christian life. She was a "tender
heart" who was easily touched by the needs of others. Satan delights
in tormenting those whose natures are gentle and tenderhearted.
Without the Word of God in their lives, they can be crushed by the
oppressive weight of the tormentor and give in to his demonic suggestion that everyone would be better off without them. On March 26,
1982, my precious mother took her own life. Two years later my
father died of diabetes and heart disease.

I'm sure you're no stranger to the pain suffered at the loss of a
loved one. In the case of suicide or murder, anger and shock combine
with grief and an overwhelming sense of loss. How can we forgive
someone who has destroyed the life God gave them? How can we forgive the person who has taken the life of someone we loved? How can
you forgive that person who hurt you so deeply?

We forgive in obedience to the Lord the same way we received forgiveness from Him—by faith. At first, forgiving others by myself was

too difficult for me. I couldn't let go of them or the pain. During this struggle, my emotions seemed to cry out, *I've been hurt! They did this to me, and they need to suffer for it! How can I forgive them?* A wise woman said to me, "If you can't forgive them yourself, ask God to forgive them through you."

One by one I held up each name on my list to the Lord. For those I couldn't bring myself to forgive, I said, "Lord, please forgive this person through me." In His gentle, patient way the Lord reminded me, *I have already forgiven them. Let go.* Oh, the tears! And finally— the freedom.

I had written more than 40 names on my forgiveness list. (Talk about holding resentments!) I even included institutions and groups of people I felt I needed to forgive for hurting me in some way. Whether the hurts were intentional or not, real or imagined, I stepped out in faith to forgive, and the Lord took me the rest of the way. I also forgave myself.

Making Music with Bruised Reeds

> *"A bruised reed He will not break, and a smoldering wick He will not snuff out."* [3]

We often feel too battered, bruised, and broken to ever be used by God. When a craftsman makes a musical instrument, he discards bruised reeds for perfect ones—but not the Lord. Any housewife in old Jerusalem knew if her oil lamp had smoking flax, it had to be doused and thrown out immediately. Its noxious fumes and black smoke meant it was good for nothing. The Lord looks at the smoldering remains of our past and says, "I can use that to help her be a blessing to someone else." Our God is so good to us, giving us "beauty for ashes." [4]

My friend, forgive, let go, and let God be God over everything in your life—even your pain. He will take the wounded heart you give Him and strengthen it into a heart of compassion to bring healing and deliverance to others. Jesus was *moved* with compassion. [5] Compassion is active. It doesn't sit by the sidelines in self-centered seclusion; it gets involved. Compassion is similar to empathy, and the word literally means "to suffer together." By God's grace, forgiveness transports you from pain to freedom.

Once you forgive, you will experience a breakthrough in your prayer life. Unforgiveness hinders our faith, but forgiveness frees our faith because faith works by love.[6] Walking in forgiveness is walking in the spirit of love, for God *is* love![7]

Bringing It Home

In this chapter I learned…

1. _____

2. _____

3. _____

I can start doing this better today:_____

_____

Lord, I ask You to help me _____

_____

7

Stress: America's Number One Health Problem

Anxiety in the heart of man causes depression,
but a good word makes it glad.

Proverbs 12:25

According to the American Institute of Stress, stress is America's number one health problem. It's estimated that 75 to 90 percent of all visits to doctors are for stress-related problems. Today's stresses tend to be more dangerous than those of the past because they primarily stem from psychological threats rather than physical.

God originally designed our bodies to have a stress response for positive reasons:

- Heart rate and blood pressure go up, increasing the flow of blood to the brain and improving decision making.
- Blood sugar rises, furnishing more fuel for energy.
- Blood is redirected from the digestive system to the large muscles of the arms and legs, providing more strength or greater speed for getting away from danger.
- Blood clotting occurs more quickly, preventing blood loss from injuries.

However, we do not usually experience stress from an occasional confrontation with a wild animal or a hostile warrior but rather from a host of emotional threats like getting stuck in traffic and having arguments with family members, coworkers, or customers. Unfortunately, our bodies can still react with these same stress responses, which are not only no longer useful but even potentially damaging and deadly. We can easily see how stress contributes to hypertension, strokes, heart attacks, diabetes, ulcers, neck or low back pain, and a host of other "diseases of civilization."

What Causes Stress?

Physical and emotional problems are the most common causes of stress. Other factors include perfectionism, work addiction, insomnia, and work-related or marriage-related problems. Dietary causes include too much sugar, caffeine, and alcohol, as well as vitamin depletion caused by a poor diet. Handling stress when symptoms first appear seems to be a key to avoiding the destruction high stress can cause.

Physical Helps

Eating more whole foods and completely eliminating sugar, soft drinks, and caffeine from my diet have helped my body handle stress more effectively. Sugar and caffeine burden the adrenal glands. These small glands just over the kidneys secrete hormones to help you cope with physical and emotional stress. When the adrenal glands are overtaxed, however, they are unable to function at their best, resulting in higher stress levels.

To decrease the stress of getting food on the table day after day, invite the family to become a part of the meal preparation process. Make menu planning, cooking, and setting the table family activities to avoid the last-minute stress of wondering what to do for dinner. I wonder if people usually order fast food simply to escape the anxiety of last-minute dinner decisions.

Dietary supplement support for stress relief includes Adrenal Fuel by NatraTech's Dr. Len Lopez; the amino acids GABA (gamma-aminobutyric acid), glutamine, glycine, lysine, and taurine; and herbs such as valerian, St. John's wort, and kava-kava. For more supplement suggestions to handle stress, please see www.BasicSteps.info.

Exercise lowers stress levels, as do the PraiseMoves postures (see chapter 9). Even a ten-minute walk can do wonders to clear the head and help your body let go of tension.

The fragrances of essential oils in a warm bath are wonderfully relaxing after a long day. Try a bath with six to ten drops of lavender essential oil or two to four drops of chamomile. Light some candles, unwind, and read a devotional book. Ahhhh...

Your mind and body need rest to perform at their peak levels, so seven to nine hours of sleep each night is also important. Continually forcing your body to work on inadequate sleep is hard on the immune system and can lead to stress, mental fatigue, and illness.

Stop, Tune, and Turn

Daily prayer, exercise, and dietary changes will make a big difference in your ability to handle stress. I've found prayer and spending time in the Word especially helpful in *avoiding* some of the stresses people face. When you know for a certainty that your times are in His hand,[1] and that Jesus Christ has redeemed you from the curse of the law[2] (poverty, sickness, and spiritual death), you have peace that comes directly from God. And what the Prince of Peace gives you, the world cannot take away.

Yes, I can lose my peace if I choose to give it away and give in to the pressure of circumstances and the enemy. Yet if I will *stop* focusing on the world's yakking and *tune* in to God, I can *turn* on my heels and go the opposite direction, entering His rest and finding peace. In this place of peace, we are quiet enough to hear from God and receive wisdom to solve the problems facing us.

Seven hundred years before Jesus came to earth, the Holy Spirit inspired the prophet Isaiah to write about God's suffering Servant, who would take upon Himself the sins of mankind. The Amplified Bible's interpretation of Isaiah 53:5 helped me understand that when Jesus bore the sins of the whole world, He took upon Himself our physical, mental, and emotional pains, stresses, and sicknesses as well. "The chastisement [needful to obtain] peace and well-being for us was upon Him, and with the stripes [that wounded] Him we are healed and made whole."

One Bible teacher told me that the crown of thorns on Jesus' brow reminded her that He bore our mental and emotional stress and anguish. It's a vivid image that prompts me to remember He bore the "chastisement" of my peace (all care, stress, and anxiety), so I would be insulting the Lord by retaining what He bore for me. We need humility to cast our cares on the Lord. "Therefore humble yourselves under the mighty hand of God, that He may exalt you in due time, casting all your care upon Him, for He cares for you."[3] Pride says, "Never mind, God. I'll handle this one myself." That kind of thinking and behavior is a prescription for stress and anxiety.

Scriptural Medicine for Freedom from Stress

"Be anxious for nothing, but in everything by prayer and supplication, with thanksgiving, let your requests be made known to God; and the peace of God, which surpasses all understanding, will guard your hearts and minds through Christ Jesus."[4]

Quoting Paul's affirmation to the Philippians is a powerful stress buster. Apply it to yourself right now: "I am anxious for nothing, but in everything by prayer and supplication, with thanksgiving, I make my requests to God; and the peace of God, which surpasses all understanding, guards my heart and mind through Christ Jesus."

Now make your prayer request. Prayer is talking to God. Supplication is humbly asking for and expecting His help. Once you've asked, rejoice! That's thanksgiving. You don't need to continually beg and whine. If you made a request to your heavenly Father according to His Word, He heard you the first time, and "we know we have the petitions that we have asked of Him."[5] Just keep thanking and praising Him that your prayer is answered—regardless of what the circumstances look like.

Well, Laurette, that's easy for you to say, you may be thinking. *You don't know the pressure I'm under.* No, I don't know the difficulties you face, but I do know the stresses the Lord has brought me through. I know that when we go to Him with the big problems and the small ones, He *will* make a way out of the mess even when there seems to be no way out. The times I have been the most stressed and frustrated were the times I was "playing God" and trying to work things out on my own.

The Holy Spirit will sometimes prompt you to surrender at a deeper level than ever before. If you thrive on control, this is one of the most gut-wrenching things you will ever do—and the most freeing.

I thought I had come to the end of myself for the first and last time on April 1, 1987, when I cried out to God and surrendered my life to Jesus Christ. I was mistaken. I have come to places of surrender all along the trail since then. For example, in November 2002, I sensed discomfort in my spirit for months—like rubbing against sandpaper. I wondered if I was going in the wrong direction. Nothing was working. At the leading of the Lord, I had put PraiseMoves and the one-woman musical drama *Great Women of the Bible* on the shelf for a year until I was certain He wanted me to present them to the public.

After much internal struggle I finally surrendered—again! Why does it take some of us so long to give up? I came to the place where it didn't matter if I ever acted, wrote, or sang another song (all things I love). If it wasn't God's will for me, I would have none of it. *Now I can use you,* I sensed Him say in my heart.

We sometimes say we're waiting on God, but I think He's often waiting on us.

Within two months I was teaching PraiseMoves classes, booking meetings, and rehearsing for the opening of *Great Women of the Bible.* Time seemed to be compressed, and I was able to get an enormous amount of work done in a short amount of time. Talk about a stress reliever! When you give God complete control of your life, He will give you favor, open doors no man can shut, and shut doors no man can open.

What is the one thing you haven't entrusted to the Lord yet? What are you still trying to figure out or make happen? Write it here:_____ _____. Now, what situation is inviting you to worry (to meditate on the destructive plans of the enemy)? Write it here: _____.

Do you think the One who spoke the universe into existence through His Word[6] and formed you in your mother's womb has a few answers you may not have considered? Why not come to Him with those situations right now? The more baggage you discard, the lighter you will become emotionally, mentally, *and* physically. The more you give of yourself to God, the more peace, health, and godly fitness you will enjoy.

Please pray this with me:

> *Heavenly Father, forgive me for not completely trusting You. Without You I can do nothing, but with You all things are possible. I give everything to You, Lord—all my*

dreams, mistakes, opinions, fears, abilities, and desires. I especially give You _____
(name the situations and concerns). *I don't know what's right for me, but You do. I surrender every part of my life to You, knowing You will give me the abundant life You want me to live in return. Your way is far better than anything I could possibly figure out myself. If You're not in it, Lord, I don't want it. Your Word says that when I delight myself in You, You will give me the desires of my heart.*[7] *Thank You, Father, for lining up my desires with Your perfect will. Your will be done in my life, in Jesus' name. Amen.*

"There remains therefore a rest for the people of God. For he who has entered His rest has himself also ceased from his works as God did from His. Let us therefore be diligent to enter that rest."[8]

Bringing It Home

In this chapter I learned...

1. _____

2. _____

3. _____

I can start doing this better today: _____

_____

Lord, I ask You to help me _____

_____

Step Three

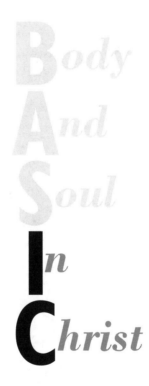

Body
And
Soul

In
Christ

8

Prayer, Praise, and Fasting:
God's Power Tools

Prayer

Prayer is talking to God. It is little more than that—with one addition. Prayer also involves *listening* to God. Like any good conversation, prayer includes the give-and-take of two-way communication. How long would your loved ones tolerate your doing all the talking during your conversations with one another?

For some reason, most of us tend to think prayer is a one-way street. We talk (or whine) to God about our problems and then spend the rest of the day worrying and trying to figure out solutions ourselves. Then we gripe when God doesn't seem to answer our prayers. Could He even get a word in edgewise?

If you had been one of Jesus' disciples when He walked the earth, what are some of the things you would have asked Him? In the biblical account, none of the disciples asked Jesus to tell them how He raised the dead, calmed the sea, or caused a fish to be caught with a coin in its mouth. They didn't ask how He multiplied the loaves and fishes or walked on the water. But they did ask, "Lord, teach us to pray."[1] They realized something powerful happened whenever Jesus went off by Himself to pray. Jesus answered their request by giving them what we refer to as The Lord's Prayer, recorded in Luke 11:2-4 and Matthew 6:9-13.

In chapter 4 we looked at "A Daily Walk with the Lord's Prayer." You can use that same scriptural formula for your quiet prayer time. It's a great way to fellowship with the Lord, praise, pray the priorities, and *listen*.

Over the years I've used several formulas for prayer that involve acronyms to help me remember the steps to effective prayer: ACTS (Adoration, Confession, Thanksgiving, Supplication), CATS (Confession, Adoration, Thanksgiving, Supplication), and PART (Pardon, Adoration, Request, Thanksgiving—or Praise, Admit, Request, Thank). These are wonderful formulas to help us keep on track with our prayers, but I wanted an acronym that would include a step to remind me to listen to God. I came up with two: The first is CARAT (the unit of weight for precious stones—and prayer is precious!). The second acronym is RARE.

CARAT (Confess, Adore, Request, Attend, Thank)

Confess: Wipe the slate clean first thing if you have unconfessed sin. Ask God to forgive you. You do not need to confess things you did *before* you accepted Christ. He has removed those things "as far as the east is from the west."[2] He blots out our mistakes and forgets our sins for His own sake.[3] What a mighty and merciful God we serve!

Adore: Praise Him with your whole heart and your voice. What if you don't feel like it? That's why Hebrews refers to a "sacrifice of praise!"[4] Your flesh would rather go back to bed, but you're not going to be led by your flesh anymore, right?

To help you get started, read one of the Psalms of David aloud, such as Psalm 34, 95, 96, 98, 100, 103, 121, 148, or 150. Then use your own words as well to tell your heavenly Father how much you love Him.

Request: Ask God to meet your needs and the needs of others. Here are some ideas: Pray for our leaders (that they hear and follow God's guidance and that godly men and women be placed in positions of influence), for our nation and your community (for protection, prosperity, and a turn from evil), and for persecuted Christians and issues in the news. Instead of clucking our tongues at what we see on the news, let's pray for these people and situations. Pray for your pastor, church leaders, and other churches. Pray for services held at your church (that the lost will be saved and that believers will grow in faith). Pray for friends, family, and yourself.

If you are unsure how to pray for others, go to the Word. For example, if you are praying for a family member's healing from cancer, look at Deuteronomy 28:61 and Galatians 3:13. Blessings and curses were associated with following or breaking the Law as given to Moses for the Hebrews. The blessings for observing God's command-ments are listed in Deuteronomy 28:1-14, and the curses of disobe-dience are listed in verses 15-68. Jesus Christ saved and redeemed us from the curse of the Law, which included a host of sicknesses, plagues, and devastations. Obviously, a number of sicknesses and dis-eases today were unknown thousands of years ago. Thankfully, God thinks of everything! Verse 61 covers every conceivable illness including cancer, AIDS, multiple sclerosis, Parkinson's disease, schiz-ophrenia, and diseases that have not even been identified yet. This passage from Deuteronomy says, "*Every* sickness and *every* plague, which is not written in this Book of the Law, will the LORD bring upon you." (The Hebrew could literally be rendered, "...will the Lord allow to *ascend* upon you"[5]—we know God is not the author of disease.) However, Galatians 3:13 reminds us that "Christ has redeemed us from the curse of the law, having become a curse for us."

You might pray, *Father, according to Deuteronomy 28:61, cancer is under the curse of the law, and according to Galatians 3:13, Jesus Christ redeemed us from the curse of the law. So, Father, I thank You that _____ is redeemed from cancer.* If the people for whom you are praying are believers, I would share those two Scriptures with them and ask them to repeat them aloud over and over to build their faith. This is not a magic formula or what Jesus called "vain repetitions,"[6] for you are asking them to feed on the truth of the Word of God for themselves to build their faith. Speaking God's Word is certainly not vain repetition. God's words "are life to those that find them, and health to all their flesh."[7] The word for health in Hebrew is *marpê*, which literally means "medicine." You can consider speaking the Word over your body as taking daily doses of God's medicine! Lis-tening to Scriptures read to soothing music is also helpful.

Attend: The King James Version of Proverbs 4:20 says, "My son, *attend* to my words; incline thine ear unto my sayings." When we attend to God, we pay attention to His words in Scripture and wait upon Him to receive further revelation and guidance. Listen for His "still small voice."[8] The Holy Spirit or your own spirit may quicken a Scripture to your remembrance for you to meditate. I strongly recommend having a journal with you to write down ideas and guidance as the Lord directs you. The answer to many a perplexing situation has come to me as I sat quietly waiting on the Lord, pen in hand.

Thanksgiving: Jesus said, "Whatever things you ask when you pray, believe that you receive them, and you will have them."[9] How do you respond when you receive something wonderful? Thanking God for answering your prayers is just the sensible thing to do. Some may wonder, *Why? How do I know that God will answer my prayers?* If you are praying according to God's will (His Word in the Bible), you have His promise that He hears and *will* answer your prayer. "Now this is the confidence that we have in Him, that if we ask anything according to His will, He hears us. And if we know that He hears us, whatever we ask, we know that we have the petitions that we have asked of Him."[10]

You can be confident that God hears and answers prayer, so rejoice! Dance in advance—even before you see the outward manifestation of the answer to your prayer. We're to keep our focus on the unseen spiritual truths instead of the physical circumstances. "For the things which are seen are temporary, but the things which are not seen are eternal."[11] Things come to life in the realm of the spirit before we see them physically. That's why the writer of the book of Hebrews calls faith "the *evidence* of things not seen."[12] Jesus told us to believe that we receive the answer to prayer "when you pray," not after it has appeared physically. Thank your heavenly Father for answered prayer. You can even get excited about it!

RARE (Repent, Adore, Request, Expect)

Repent: This is the same step as *Confess* listed above. Repent means to be truly sorry for wrongdoing and making a complete 180-degree turn away from that sin. No, it doesn't mean feeling sorry you got caught (but you knew that)!

Adore: This step is explained above.

Request: This step is explained above.

Expect: Expect to hear from God. Expect Him to answer your prayer. Expect to receive all you need to do all God has called you to do. Expectation is "sit on the edge of your seat" excitement. The ticket is in your hand, you're eagerly ready to go, and you're just waiting to hear your name called—and you're next! That's faith-based expectation.

This step is a combination of the *Attend* and *Thanksgiving* steps above. Listen expectantly for God's guidance. Jesus, speaking of Himself as our Shepherd, said, "The sheep follow him, for they know his voice."[13]

Mountain-Moving Prayer

The Lord gave us the perfect prayer outline in Mark 11 for removing mountains in our life. Mountains are situations and conditions that stand between us and the fulfillment of God's best for us. Mountains standing in your way can be things such as lack, debt, or a bad credit report. A mountain can be a physical, emotional, or mental limitation, a relationship challenge, or a job situation. Even if the mountain in your way appears to be a certain person, the enemy is not that person. "For we do not wrestle against flesh and blood, but against principalities, against powers, against the rulers of the darkness of this age, against spiritual hosts of wickedness in the heavenly places."[14]

Have you noticed that the enemy always attacks you in the area of your greatest gift? For me, fear of people and worry over what they thought about me was a mountain that stood in the way of the gift of communication the Lord gave me. I had a desire to act, write, speak—to communicate in any form—but fear kept me from taking action. I had to resist that mountainous "spirit of fear" that was not from God but from Satan. In the Scripture in which Paul mentions the spirit of fear (2 Timothy 1:6-7), he exhorts Timothy to "stir up the gift of God" within him. He reminds Timothy, "God has not given us a spirit of fear, but of power and of love and of a sound mind." God has given *you* power, love, and a sound mind (also translated "discipline" and "self-control").

If you are afraid to express the desire of your heart, the enemy is using the spirit of fear against you. He knows about the lives you will touch and win to God by expressing your God-given gifts and talents, so he will try his utmost to stop you. He'll say things such as *You can't do it. You're just being conceited. No one in the family has ever done anything like that. People will talk about you. Who do you think you are?*

You may even have become so accustomed to that negative, accusatory voice that you think it's your own voice saying, *I'm scared. I can't do that. What will people think?* My friend, if Satan *can* stop you, he will. *You* are the one who decides whether he can or not. Remember that "he walks about *like* a roaring lion, seeking whom he may devour."[15] He's not a roaring lion; he's only sounds like one. His teeth were knocked out by Jesus. *You* decide if he may try to devour you or not.

The temptation is to talk about the mountain that stands in our way. Jesus, however, did not tell us to talk *about* the mountain. He told us to talk *to* the mountain. I've used this method of prayer for almost 15 years now and have noticed an interesting thing. For each goal set and prayer prayed using this outline, one of three things has happened: It has come to pass, it is in the process of coming to pass, or it is no longer important to me. That's the power of focused, mountain-moving prayer! I believe it will be a blessing to you too.

Use the template that follows to list the mountains facing you, your requests and goals, and people you need to forgive. Then read the entire outline aloud during your prayer time. Change it from time to time as you see the mountains moved and prayers answered. God's Word works! Speak it aloud daily.

Mark 11:22-25: A Template for Mountain-Moving Prayer

Have faith in God.
Lord, I believe in You.

For assuredly, I say to you, whoever says to this mountain...
These are the mountains I am facing:

1. _____

2. _____

3. _____

4. _____

5. _____

… *"Be removed and be cast into the sea," and does not doubt in his heart, but believes that those things he says will be done, he will have whatever he says.*

I say to these mountains, "Be removed and be cast into the sea!" I do not doubt in my heart, but I believe those things I say will be done. I know I will have whatever I say.

These are my prayer requests and goals:

1. _____

2. _____

3. _____

4. _____

5. _____

Therefore I say to you, whatever things you ask when you pray, believe that you receive them, and you will have them.

I believe I receive those things I ask for when I pray. I trust that I will have them.

And whenever you stand praying, if you have anything against anyone, forgive him, that your Father in heaven may also forgive you your trespasses. But if you do not forgive, neither will your Father in heaven forgive your trespasses.

These are the people I forgive:

1. _____

2. _____

3. _____

4. _____

5. _____

Now praise the Lord for answered prayer! He is faithful.

The Power of Praise

We looked at praise in the *Adore* steps above, but now we can add something more. Psalm 22:3 tells us that God *inhabits* the praises of His people. Some people describe this by saying that the Lord comes down from heaven and sits on the throne created by our praise. Isn't that a remarkable image? Could God sit comfortably on the throne of *your* praise? Halfhearted praise is more like a two-legged stool. Yikes!

You can sing and speak praises to God throughout the day. Memorize portions of the Psalms that exalt the virtues of God. Meditate on them and speak them aloud—to the Lord. You can maintain a sweet communion with Him as you work, drive, or shop. When you are praising God, your mind is off your problems and on the One who can solve your problems. Isaiah said, "You will keep him in perfect peace, whose mind is stayed on You."[16]

Miracles at Midnight

Paul and Silas knew about the power of praise. Whipped, beaten, and chained together in a cold, filthy dungeon, these two men were not in ideal praise circumstances—or were they? "And at midnight Paul and Silas prayed, and sang praises unto God: and the prisoners heard them."[17] They were praying and singing praises loud enough for other prisoners to hear them, so they certainly weren't mumbling halfhearted choruses of "Kumbaya."

The very next verse reads: "And suddenly there was a great earthquake, so that the foundations of the prison were shaken: and immediately all the doors were opened, and every one's bands were loosed." No foe can withstand the presence of the living God. Prisons of fear and pain cannot hold the daughter of God who throws her head back and lifts her heart, hands, and voice in praise of her heavenly Father.

Praise renews your mind, lifts your emotions, and puts you in vital contact with the Lord. I've been in the middle of a trying situation and decided to start praising God instead of worrying. I remind myself that Jesus is Lord over my life. I thank Him that He's working it all out—and He does!

Prayer and praise are two of God's dynamic "power tools." The third is fasting.

Fasting: The Bondage Breaker

God designed fasting "to loose the bonds of wickedness, to undo the heavy burdens, to let the oppressed go free, and...break every yoke." He calls this "the fast that I have chosen."[18]

For many years I would not fast. I was convinced I could not fast. The idea of going without food for even one day was beyond my grasp. Part of the reason I wasn't obedient to Jesus' words *"when* you fast..."[19] was that I was afraid I couldn't do it. I thought I'd cheat, fall into sin, and be hopelessly lost. Well, maybe that's a bit of an exaggeration, but most of my excuses for not fasting were fear-based hyperbole.

The Bible refers to fasting more than 80 times. The word *fasting* appears 30 more times than the word *food.* Fasting is a spiritual discipline whereby you deliberately deny the body's physical desire for food in order to devote yourself to prayer and communion with the Lord.

The Bible includes examples of fasts that lasted one day, three days, seven days, ten days, twenty-one days, and forty days.

A cautionary note: Anyone desiring to go on a fast for longer than three days should consult first with his or her health care provider. Those taking medication should see their physician before starting a fast. Please do not fast if you are pregnant or lactating. Toxins are eliminated during fasts, and we don't want a baby ingesting toxins into his or her little body.

Reasons to Fast

1. to break down prison walls (physical, emotional, and mental)
2. to break the power of the lusts of the flesh (greed, gluttony, covetousness, and perversion)
3. for clearer guidance and direction from the Lord on specific issues
4. to intercede for others
5. to strengthen your relationship with God
6. to debilitate the power of the enemy against you
7. to overcome temptation, confusion, and frustration
8. for physical cleansing and healing
9. to seek new focus and direction for your life from God
10. to walk in greater strength and victory in every area of your life

I have found fasting to be a vital part of overcoming food addictions (sugar, caffeine, and overeating), destroying mental strongholds (negative patterns of thought), defeating the lusts of the flesh, and receiving clear direction from God when unsure what path to take.

Fasting doesn't win points with God or enable Him to hear your prayers any better. It *does* quiet your flesh and mind to help you hear from God more clearly. If your carnal nature has been in control, fasting will enable your spirit (the real you) to gain the upper hand— if you fast as to the Lord. Fasting without prayer yields limited results beyond the loss of a few pounds (that you'll quickly gain back when the fast is over). Fasting *with* prayer breaks strongholds at the root of overeating, depression, or whatever bondage is holding you back.

How to Fast

Plan ahead of time when you will fast. Begin by fasting one meal or for one day and devoting the time to prayer instead of eating. When I fast, I like to have a particular prayer subject or reason why I'm fasting. During meal times, instead of eating I devote that time to praise, prayer, and reading the Word.

I recommend beginning a fast when you can be at home without the everyday stresses of the workplace. If you work at home, pick a time when you know you could rest if you needed to do so.

For those new to fasting, I recommend a fruit and vegetable juice fast instead of a water-only fast. You can get a good, reasonably priced juicer from your local health food or department store. If you must use store-bought juices at first, get organic juices whenever possible. Fruit juices should be diluted with water due to their high fruit sugar content.

Drink at least two quarts (64 ounces) of pure, clean water every day in addition to the fruit and vegetable juices. Water helps remove toxins from your system.

Juice Fast Recipes

Wash all fruits and vegetables (preferably organic), and run them through your juicer. Follow these recipes or create your own!

1. Wake-Up Call: a small handful of parsley with four to five carrots (half apple optional)

2. Pinkie Lady: a peeled pink grapefruit with one apple (core removed)

3. Green Power Drink: a handful of spinach, three kale leaves, three sprigs parsley, six carrots, and one scoop of concentrated greens powder (I use Ultimate Living's Green Miracle—see www.BasicSteps.info)

4. Popeye n' Olive Oyl: a big handful of spinach and six tall, skinny carrots

5. Sweet 'n' Sassy: four carrots, a handful of parsley, half an apple, and two celery stalks

6. Can't Elope? Oh, Honey Do: half a cantaloupe, half a honeydew melon, six strawberries

7. Kiss Me, Kale: two kale leaves, a handful of spinach, two tomatoes, one stalk celery

8. Orange Blossom Special: two or three peeled oranges, one apple, a quarter-inch slice of ginger root

9. Berry-Grape Sparkle: two cups each strawberries, blueberries, and grapes. Add ice and sparkling water.

10. Feel the Beet: one half large beet, two or three apples (core removed), two or three stalks celery

11. Spicy Lemonade: one (or one-half) lemon, one teaspoon pure maple syrup or packet of stevia, one or two dashes of cayenne pepper, six to eight ounces of water. Serve hot or cold.

For added nutrition, add a concentrated greens powder to any of the juices, or simply mix it with water. See www.BasicSteps.info for more recipes and suggestions.

Coming Off a Fast

Come off a fast *slowly!* This is not a play on words. Ending a fast by eating small amounts of solid food is extremely important. When your digestive system has had a lighter load for a few days, dumping a big meal on it would not only be a shock but could also prove extremely harmful to your health. Reintroduce food gradually. The longer your fast, the more time you'll need to adjust to solid food.

Break your fast with a *small* amount of fresh fruit or vegetables—never meat, dairy, or processed foods. I hope that you'll find these foods less desirable than before. A fast is a great way to overcome our flesh's cravings for heavier, processed fare. Your system has had a cleansing, so you should find the taste and fragrance of natural foods more pleasing.

You can actually train yourself to desire purer foods this way. God used fasting to break my addictions to sugar and caffeine. I remember when I could not have imagined passing by a sugary dessert without having one—or two! Now by the grace of God and the strength He's given me through prayer and fasting, I'm able to say, "No, thank you."

If you have fasted less than three days, break the fast by eating small amounts of fresh non-citrus fruit (such as apples, watermelon, grapes, or berries) at meal times and a small fresh vegetable salad for dinner. Continue to drink two quarts of water throughout the day. You may continue drinking several juice drinks as well. On the second day you can add vegetables and grains, but be aware that your body will likely need less food than before. Be sensitive to your "full signal," and do not overeat. Ask the Lord to help you end your fast with grace so you will not nullify the health benefits you've achieved.

To end fasts of three days and longer, add solid food more gradually. Continue to drink two quarts of water and several fresh juice drinks per day. Eat small amounts of fruit until dinner of the second day, when you can have a bowl of freshly made vegetable soup (not canned). Add a salad or small baked potato (no butter, cheese, or sour cream) for dinner. Have a slice of sprouted grain bread (like Ezekiel 4:9 bread) or a small amount of brown rice.

On the fourth day you can add one or two ounces of free-range poultry (without hormones and other chemicals). Be prayerfully careful *not* to overeat during this time.

By the fifth day you can begin following the food plan outlined in earlier chapters (following the Mediterranean model). Continue drinking two quarts of water and a fresh juice drink or two. Your eyes should be absolutely sparkling by now!

Tips for Fasting

1. Eat lightly and include more fruits and vegetables for a day or two before your fast. You will be extremely

uncomfortable starting a fast if your body is full of large amounts of processed foods it is trying to eliminate.

2. Take a walk outdoors and exercise lightly while fasting. Breathe deeply, swing your arms, and put a smile on your face.

3. If you feel the need, take a gentle herbal laxative tea in the evening before bedtime. This is also a good thing to drink the night before a fast begins.

4. Dry brush your skin and bathe daily to remove impurities from pores. Brush your teeth and your tongue (which will be coated as toxins are released). That will help control bad breath.

5. Rest. Be sure to get seven to nine hours of sleep a night. If you need to nap during the day, go right ahead. I have to remind myself that's okay!

6. Do not ingest caffeine, sugar, alcohol, or artificial ingredients or chemicals. Please do not smoke!

7. Realize that symptoms of headache, coated tongue, weakness, and cold are not uncommon. The caffeine withdrawal headache can be a real humdinger, but hang in there. By the second day it's usually gone, and you'll begin feeling better than you have in years (I sure did!).

8. Drink water or a juice drink to overcome hunger pangs. Usually the juice drinks are so satisfying you won't feel much discomfort.

9. How often should you fast? Some people fast one day a week or half a day twice a week. Some fast two or three days a month. Others fast one day a week and then fast for three weeks several times a year. There are no definite rules. Just start slowly and follow the leading of the Lord.

Remember that you are fasting as to the Lord. Make the most of this special time by keeping a journal to record new insights and answers to prayer the Lord gives you. Press in to know Him more intimately than you ever have before. The times of fasting I have experienced have been life changers for me. Strongholds and addictions were broken. I received guidance, and attained a closer communion with the Lord since I decided to put away my hunger for food and rekindle my hunger for *Him*.

May He grant you all your heart can hold during these times of precious communion.

Bringing It Home

In this chapter I learned...

1. _____

2. _____

3. _____

I can start doing this better today: _____

_____

Lord, I ask You to help me _____

_____

9

PraiseMoves: The Christian Alternative to Yoga

As I mentioned in the introduction, I was introduced to yoga as a little girl when my mother began watching a daily yoga exercise program on television. This opened the door to New Age mysticism, yoga, and a host of other deceptive mind-sets and religious practices until I became a Christian in 1987.

But wait, you may be thinking. *Yoga isn't a religion; it's just an exercise technique, isn't it?*

Since starting a PraiseMoves website a few years ago, we've had many interesting comments from Christians and non-Christians across North America and numerous foreign countries. Most have been very supportive of PraiseMoves, though a few have been defensive or antagonistic. I recently received an unsolicited e-mail from a yoga academy on the East Coast. Apparently they had been told about our www.PraiseMoves.com and about my view that yoga is more than just an exercise program. A member of the staff at the Classical Yoga Hindu Academy wrote, "Yes, all of Yoga is Hinduism. Everyone should be aware of this fact."

Others ask, "How can yoga be dangerous? Aren't physicians, chiropractors, and physiotherapists recommending yoga to their patients?" Yes, some people in the medical field have been recommending yoga to their patients suffering from arthritis, fibromyalgia, osteoporosis, stress, and a host of other ailments. A Christian chiropractor on the East Coast told me he had been recommending yoga to his patients until he learned more about the root and the fruit of yoga. "I kept having this recurring dream," he told me. "I saw the Lord, and He asked me why I led so many of His sheep down the wrong path into yoga. I'd wake up in a cold sweat, remembering the Scripture about causing one of God's little ones to stumble—that it would be better if a millstone were hung around that person's neck and he were cast into the sea. I realized I had to see if something else was out there. I did an Internet search and found PraiseMoves."

I'm grateful that he and other chiropractors have found PraiseMoves to have many of the physical benefits of yoga without the spiritual and mental baggage that goes along with it.

Some Christians claim, "Oh, I'm not doing the meditation stuff, just the yoga exercises. It's relaxing." Some have told me they only practice hatha yoga. "Lighten up! It's just exercise," they tell me. But hatha yoga is what I was involved in.

The number of Christians who have turned to yoga for stress relief and to improve their bodies has increased over the years. Popular chain stores offer yoga mats, videos, and other yoga paraphernalia. "Yoga must be okay—it's even at 'Wally-World!' " While seemingly commonplace in mainstream America, many Christians struggle with yoga's undercurrents of Hindu and New Age mysticism.

One precious young lady told me, "During my first yoga class, there was a check in my spirit that I shouldn't be doing this, so I stopped."

I am reminded of the Scriptures "For as many as are led by the Spirit of God, these are the sons of God" and "The sheep follow Him, for they know His voice."[1]

Most yoga practitioners will argue that yoga is not a religion but a science. A light scratching of the surface, however, reveals not only a religion but a life-encompassing (mind-numbing) philosophy as well. Forgive the hyperbole—this comes from my own experiences during 22 years of involvement with yoga and the New Age movement.

What would you say to the man who insists he's a "Christian Buddhist"? Would you say he's fooling himself? Similarly, "Christian yoga" is an oxymoron. It is not Christian. It's yoga.

Yoga actually means "union with god" or "to yoke." One goal pervades all systems of yoga: obtaining oneness with the universe or universal mind (a New Age ideology) known as Brahman or "enlight-enment" in Hinduism and as the state of Nirvana in Buddhism.

Yoga's breathing techniques *(pranayama)* may seem stress-relieving, yet they can open one to psychic influences, as does the customary relaxation period at the end of a yoga session. I remember numerous instances of "traveling outside my body" during yoga relaxation periods. I wonder who—or what—checked in when I checked out?

According to Swami Vishnudevananda, one of yoga's most influential leaders, hatha yoga "prescribes physical methods to begin...so that the student can manipulate the mind more easily as he advances, attaining communication with one's higher self."[2] The student seems to be manipulated as well. Yoga's "least religious" form, hatha yoga, influences one's spiritual life as unmistakably as any one of the dozens of other yoga techniques.

Yoga enthusiasts claim that physical and mental disciplines bring about union with God. According to Maharishi Mahesh Yogi (once associated with the Beatles), meditation "brings us more ability for achieving something through right means, and very easily a sinner comes out of the field of sin and becomes a virtuous man."[3] Oh, really?

The Bible tells us, "For all have sinned; all fall short of God's glorious standard. Yet now God in His gracious kindness declares us not guilty. He has done this *through Christ Jesus,* who has freed us by taking away our sins.... We are made right with God when we believe that Jesus shed His blood, sacrificing His life for us."[4]

PraiseMoves Is Born

Shortly after becoming a Christian in 1987, I discovered some of the things I used to enjoy were now extremely distasteful to me—especially anything involving metaphysics or New Age thought. Yoga, with its physical exercises, meditation, and spiritual practices, became part of the past for me. I eventually learned I could meditate—on the Word of God, that is! No more focusing on "awakening" my chakras, chanting mantras, or raising my kundalini energy to stimulate my "higher self" and unite with "universal mind."

On February 25, 2001, I had just finished working out with a popular exercise video diva when I began thinking and praying. Dripping with sweat, I thought, *Wouldn't it be great if there were a kinder, gentler form of exercise without all this jumping around...gentle stretches and strengthening exercises, sort of like yoga, but without the Hindu and New Age influence...?*

As I continued to ponder the idea, I thought, *What if there were something that would move us to praise God, giving Him glory, that was actually beneficial for us...a form of exercise that would move us physically to better health and flexibility while moving us spiritually to praise the Lord...PraiseMoves!*

When I asked my husband, Paul, what he thought about the idea and the name PraiseMoves, he said, "Well, praise moves God." "That's it!" I exclaimed.

For the next two years, I prayed, studied, and developed the PraiseMoves technique. Our foundation Scripture is 1 Corinthians 6:20—"For you were bought with a price; therefore glorify God in your body and in your spirit, which are God's." I hope you will discover how PraiseMoves is different from other exercise forms you may have tried. I hope it will be an answer to prayer for Christians who are looking for an alternative to yoga and a "witty invention"[5] to win the lost.

Physical Benefits of PraiseMoves

The physical benefits of PraiseMoves are similar to those of stretching and yoga exercises. The American College of Sports Medicine (ACSM) has published a position statement on flexibility outlining its benefits. It also gives basic guidelines for the minimum requirements for stretching programs. Coaches and athletes have long used flexibility training to enhance performance and prevent injury. The ACSM lists studies showing a decline in flexibility reduces physical performance, increasing injury risks. Regular stretching can reduce these risks, improving muscular performance and quality of life. Stretching may also reduce the mental and physical effects of stress and improve the function of internal organs.[6]

ACSM recommendations include a general stretching program that involves stretches for all the major muscle groups in the body. The use of static (motionless or stationary) stretching is probably the most effective form of stretching for most people. It's best to avoid ballistic (bouncing) stretches. These may harm joints or cause muscle injuries. Slow stretches (like PraiseMoves), move a joint through its full range of movement until a stretch is felt in the muscles on the side of the joint being stretched. The ACSM recommends a stretching program be performed at least two to three days a week.

What Can PraiseMoves Do?

Improve flexibility: The greater one's flexibility, the greater the range of motion. Tight muscles make tasks involving bending and lifting difficult. By keeping the body flexible, these tasks are much easier.

Assist weight loss: Improving your flexibility with PraiseMoves can help you during other forms of exercise such as walking, cycling, and strength training, thereby improving your ability to exercise with more energy, burn more calories, and lose weight.

Strengthen muscles: By improving your flexibility and strengthening your muscles with PraiseMoves, you will not only enhance your ability to perform daily tasks, you can also improve your posture, helping alleviate common aches and pains, reducing back pain, and increasing your overall sense of health and well-being.

Promote full-body stretching: Stretching your entire body helps reduce stress and tensions, leaving you feeling refreshed with increased vitality. Blood pressure and resting heart rate can drop significantly after stretching regularly. This in turn reduces your risk of cardiovascular disease, one of the leading causes of death in America.

Improve circulation: Stretching facilitates the delivery of nutrients to muscles and assists in the removal of waste products that build up in muscle tissue during exercise. Stretching helps the lymphatic system's ability to remove toxins from the body.

Support relaxation, alleviating stress: PraiseMoves includes gentle deep breathing during the postures, enhancing relaxation and flexibility. Stress causes muscles to contract, and a persistently contracted muscle becomes stiff and painful. PraiseMoves can relax stiff muscles, thus decreasing stress, promoting a peaceful disposition and a greater sense of well-being.

Help injuries to heal: Physical therapists know stretching is a vital part of rehabilitation. By stretching injured muscles gently, you can cause muscle fibers to heal more quickly with less pain and stiffness, more strength and resilience. Breast cancer survivors have used Praise-Moves to gently heal and stretch tight muscles.

Improve coordination and agility: As we become older, the importance of flexibility increases. Lack of coordination and agility is a cause of numerous injuries and accidents. By increasing flexibility, coordination, and agility, you reduce the likelihood of such injuries. There is now evidence that gentle stretches performed on a regular basis help prevent or reverse osteoporosis, actually increasing bone density and easing symptoms of menopause.

Help keep tissues healthier: Stretching encourages the release of tissue lubricants. It prevents muscle fibers from attaching to one another and inhibiting the natural fluid movement of muscles. Stretching also helps keep tissues well hydrated and more functional.

PraiseMoves strives to balance flexibility, strength, endurance, and relaxation, while spiritually "focusing on things above."

What Does a PraiseMoves Session Look Like?

PraiseMoves postures are integrated with corresponding Bible verses. For example, during the standing posture stretch The Eagle, we consider Isaiah 40:31: "But those who wait upon the LORD shall renew their strength; they shall mount up with wings like eagles, they shall run and not be weary, they shall walk and not faint." But first we warm up.

PraiseMoves' Walkin' Wisdom Warm-Ups

This is how we begin each session. Our goal is to prepare the body for the PraiseMoves workout. Muscles warm, circulation increases, and spirits rise. Walk or jog in place for 14 minutes (one mile) to upbeat contemporary Christian, praise and worship, or gospel music.

Alternate gentle, easy steps to keep things interesting. Recite several Scriptural affirmations. For example, while walking or moving to a peppy pace, say this affirmation from Ephesians 6:10: "I am strong in the Lord and the power of His might!" With the thousands of promises available in the Word of God, you have a lot of affirmations from which to choose.

Make it personal. Speak scriptural affirmations in the first person. For example: "My body is the temple of the Holy Spirit!" and "Greater is He who is in me than he who is in the world!"[7]

Note: Following our outline for the Gimme Ten Workout, you may choose to do the PraiseMoves postures after your Tuesday,

Thursday, and Saturday sessions. Your body will already be warmed up, so you won't need to do the Walkin' Wisdom Warm-Ups first.

PraiseMoves Postures

Spend the next 20 to 30 minutes practicing these gentle, effective yet *challenging* postures designed to increase flexibility and muscle strength. Soothing classical or instrumental worship music can be played during your session (or see "Resources").

Hold each posture for three to five gentle, deep breaths in and out through the nose and consider the corresponding Scripture. Your muscles will take about 30 seconds to relax and adapt to the stretch.

WWJD Meditation and Relaxation

After the postures, allow yourself to relax. Resting on the floor with your eyes closed, prayerfully consider a proverb or other portion of Scripture. Thank the Lord for this time to honor Him while exercising the temple He's given you to cherish.

All in all, PraiseMoves is an exciting workout. People often tell me they feel energized but relaxed after a workout. The body is exercised gently yet thoroughly, and all the while you are renewing your mind through the Word while "looking unto Jesus, the author and finisher of our faith."[8]

Words to the Wise

Remain relaxed throughout. Breathe deeply and gently three to five times in and out through the nose while holding each posture (or for as long as you can relax the muscles into the stretch—this may only be for a few seconds at first—building up to 30-45 seconds).

If you are healthy and accustomed to exercise, you will most likely be able to do these postures and stretches easily. However, if you have a medical condition, are pregnant, or are unsure if you should do these postures, consult your physician first.

Wear loose clothing for the PraiseMoves. Bare feet or socks are preferable. Wear running shoes during Walkin' Wisdom Warm-Ups.

Practice on a nonslip surface (you may want to get a PraiseMoves nonslip mat—see "Resources").

Exercise on an empty stomach. Keep water handy.

Start slowly. We want to *coax* the body into these postures. No forcing allowed. Feeling the stretch is good; feeling pain is not. Be patient with yourself—God is!

As you relax your muscles and extend your body into these postures, you will be lengthening your muscles, creating space in your joints and promoting freedom of movement.

Breathing Tips:

Practice breathing as deeply as you can, filling the lungs.

Breathe in and out through the nose unless otherwise directed.

Do not hold your breath in a posture. That creates tension.

When you are going into a posture, exhale. While in a posture, breathe in a deep, gentle flow. Keep your shoulders and neck relaxed.

Just before coming out of a posture, breathe in. Exhale as you gently come out of the stretch.

The Postures and the Scriptures

Keep this book in front of you so you can look at the instructions, the photos, and the corresponding Scripture for each posture.

Say the Scripture out loud or to yourself while in the posture. If the Scripture is a promise from God, make it personal! Put it in the first person and claim it for yourself and your loved ones. For example, while in The Angel posture, you may personalize Psalm 91:11 by saying, "I thank the Lord He gives His angels charge over my family and me to keep us safe in all our ways."

Pray Before You Begin

Dedicate this time to God. PraiseMoves is not something you've got to do. It's something you *get* to do. You can make this a precious time of fellowship with the Lord. Ask Him to guide you and unfold new revelations from the Scriptures as you perform these postures.

You may want to pray along these lines:

> *Heavenly Father, I thank You for the ability to exercise the body You have given me. Lord, Your Word says my body is the temple of the Holy Spirit. I choose to take good care of my body so I can be healthy and strong and full of energy to serve You better, and so I might be a blessing to my*

family, friends, and the people You bring into my life. I offer this time of exercise today, Lord, as a seed of discipline for my flesh, and as a time to draw closer to You as I meditate on Your holy Word. Thank You, Lord, for this opportunity to praise You as I move to greater levels of flexibility, strength, and health. And for all the good that comes from this, I'll be careful to give You all the praise and the glory. In Jesus' name I pray. Amen.

Walkin' Wisdom Warm-Ups

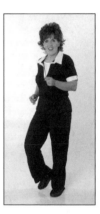

Put on some of your favorite upbeat music and walk, dance, or strut in place for 10 to 15 minutes (14 minutes is the equivalent of walking one mile at a brisk pace). Step side to side, do gentle kicks, wave your arms in circles—praise the Lord and get happy about it!

Use the affirmations that follow or ask at your local Christian bookstore for a book on "Bible Promises."

Scriptural Affirmations for Walkin' Wisdom Warm-Ups

(Repeat several of these in time to the music with feeling—and faith!)

1. I am strong in the Lord and the power of His might! (Ephesians 6:10).

2. I can do all things through Christ who strengthens me! (Philippians 4:13).

3. The joy of the Lord is my strength! (Nehemiah 8:10).

4. The Lord is the strength of my life (Psalm 27:1).

5. My body is the temple of the Holy Spirit (1 Corinthians 6:19).

6. I present my body a living sacrifice, holy and acceptable to God, which is my reasonable service (Romans 12:1).

7. (Act this one out!) I put on the whole armor of God that I may be able to stand in the evil day. I put on the

belt of truth and the breastplate of righteousness. My feet are shod with the preparation of the gospel of peace. Above all, I take the shield of faith and quench all the fiery darts of the enemy. I take the helmet of salvation and the sword of the Spirit, which is the Word of God (Ephesians 6:13-17).

8. The Word of God is a lamp for my feet and a light to my path (Psalm 119:105).

9. Wisdom is the principal thing, so I will get wisdom and understanding (Proverbs 4:7).

10. Greater is He who is in me than he who is in the world (1 John 4:4).

11. I discipline my body and bring it into subjection lest when I have preached to others I myself become disqualified (1 Corinthians 9:27).

12. I delight myself in the Lord, and He gives me the desires of my heart (Psalm 37:4).

PraiseMoves Postures

Read the instructions for each posture *before* attempting to do the pose.

Once your body is nicely warmed up, take off your shoes, place your PraiseMoves nonslip mat or a beach towel on the floor, and put on some soothing worship or classical music. Have some water to drink close at hand.

MOUNT ZION

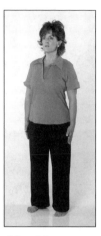

"Those who trust in the Lord *are like Mount Zion, which cannot be moved, but abides forever"* (Psalm 125:1).

Benefit: Improves posture, balance, and concentration.

- Stand with feet three or four inches apart, hands at your sides. Spread your toes apart and feel your feet in contact with the floor.

- Tighten glutes (buttocks muscles) slightly, tucking hips under, which helps take the sway out of lower back.

- Gently raise your chest up and out. Lift your body up through the rib cage, up through the neck, and through the crown of your head from the base of the skull, elongating your spine. Keep chin parallel to the floor. Keep shoulders back and neck relaxed.

- Stretch your fingers downward. Push into the floor with your feet, and lift the muscles in your calves and thighs.

- Repeat the Scripture out loud or to yourself. Breathe gently and deeply. Check your body to make sure you are not tensing up.

- Meditate (consider from every angle and reflect) on the Scripture.

- Hold the posture for three to five breaths. Relax and repeat.

THE REED

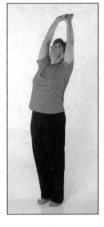

"A bruised reed He will not break, and smoking flax He will not quench" (Isaiah 42:3).

Benefit: Improves posture, balance, and flexibility of shoulders and back.

- From Mount Zion posture, bend your knees. Inhale as you sweep arms forward.
- Exhale, straightening your knees. Interlock thumbs and reach overhead.
- Breathe gently, reaching up through your waist, shoulders, and arms.
- Tighten glutes and stretch your arms slightly backward, being careful not to compress your lower back.
- Look up toward the ceiling.
- Repeat the Scripture out loud or to yourself. Breathe gently and deeply. Check your body to make sure you are not tensing up.
- Meditate on the Scripture.
- Hold the posture for three to five breaths. Relax and repeat.

THE EAGLE

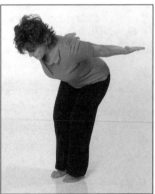

"But those who wait upon the LORD shall renew their strength; they shall mount up with wings like eagles, they shall run and not be weary, they shall walk and not faint" (Isaiah 40:31).

Benefit: Strengthens legs, back, and triceps.

- From Mount Zion posture, inhale, bending your knees slightly (do not let the knees go over toes). Bend forward with a straight back.
- Exhale, sweeping arms forward and then back like the wings of an eagle, and hold the position.

- Look down toward floor. Let lower back dip down (don't arch up). Stretch and sweep arms back, palms facing up.
- Repeat the Scripture out loud or to yourself. Breathe gently and deeply. Check your body to make sure you are not tensing up.
- Meditate on the Scripture.
- Hold the posture for three to five breaths. Relax and repeat.

THE ANGEL

"He shall give His angels charge over you, to keep you in all your ways" (Psalm 91:11).

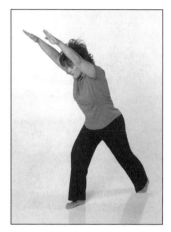

Benefit: Strengthens legs and arms, improves balance and concentration.

- Place your weight on right leg. Inhale, bringing left leg back. Point toe.
- Exhale, bending right leg. Raise arms to the front, palms down.
- Do not allow front knee to bend beyond toes.
- Bend torso forward, bringing head between arms. Reach through fingers.
- Move left toe farther back and bend right leg more.
- Repeat the Scripture out loud or to yourself. Breathe gently and deeply. Check your body to make sure you are not tensing up.
- Meditate on the Scripture.
- Hold the posture for three to five breaths. Relax and repeat with the other leg.
- *Advanced:* Raise back leg.
- Exhale and repeat with other leg.

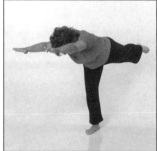

THE RAINBOW

"When I see the rainbow in the clouds, I will remember the eternal covenant between God and every living creature" (Genesis 9:16 NLT).

Benefit: Stretches spine and waist, improves balance.

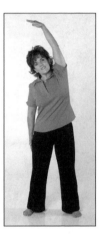

- Spread feet two feet apart, toes angled out 45 degrees.
- Inhale, raising your left arm overhead, right hand on your outer thigh. Keep abs and glutes in.
- Exhale, reach up, and bend to the right, gliding your right arm down the outside of your leg.
- Make an arc of your left arm, reaching up and back with elbow, palm facing the floor.
- Repeat the Scripture out loud or to yourself. Breathe gently and deeply. Check your body to make sure you are not tensing up.
- Meditate on the Scripture.
- Hold the posture for three to five breaths. Relax and repeat on the other side.

    •*Advanced:* Hold left wrist, pull up and to the side.

    • Repeat on the other side.

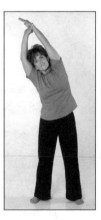

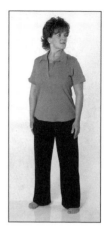

NECK STRETCHES

"Submit to God. Resist the devil and he will flee from you. Draw near to God and He will draw near to you" (James 4:7-8).

Benefit: Helps keep your neck flexible, releases tension in your neck and shoulders.

- From the Mount Zion posture, exhale looking over your right shoulder. Hold the position, breathing gently. Exhale back to center. Repeat on the left side.

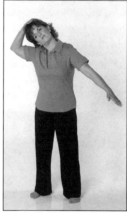

- Exhale, bringing your right ear down to your shoulder, right hand lightly on head, left arm pointing out and down to gently increase stretch. Repeat on the left side.

- Exhale, bringing your chin toward your chest.

- Keep abs and glutes in, knees soft.

- Repeat the Scripture out loud or to yourself. Breathe gently and deeply. Check your body to make sure you are not tensing up.

- Meditate on the Scripture.

- Hold the posture for three to five breaths. Exhale to release.

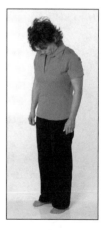

THE TALLIT (PRAYER SHAWL)

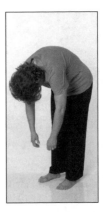

"Rejoice always, pray without ceasing, in everything give thanks; for this is the will of God in Christ Jesus for you" (1 Thessalonians 5:16-18).

Benefit: Stretches the legs and spine, relaxes the whole body.

- From Mount Zion posture, exhale, bringing chin to chest and slowly roll your body down, one vertebra at a time, arms dangling. It's okay to bend your knees slightly or rest your hands on your legs.

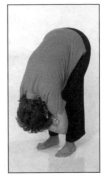

- If you can, bring your hands to floor and then fold your arms like fringes (tzitzit) on a prayer shawl. Relax, breathe.

- Meditate on the Scripture.

- Exhale, rounding up *very* slowly, pulling abs in to protect your back. Curl up one vertebra at a time. Keep your head and neck down to the very last. Ahhh…

THE STAR

"Those who are wise shall shine like the brightness of the firmament, and those who turn many to righteousness like the stars forever and ever" (Daniel 12:3).

Benefit: Strengthens legs and arms, keeps spine flexible.

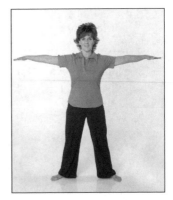

- Spread feet two to three feet apart and angled outward 45 degrees. Keep knees soft.

- Inhale, raising your arms parallel to the floor, palms down. Abs and glutes in. Reach out through your fingers and down through your feet.

- Repeat the Scripture out loud or to yourself. Breathe gently and deeply. Check your body to make sure you are not tensing up.

- Meditate upon the Scripture.

- Hold the posture for three to five breaths. Relax.

- *Advanced:* From the Star posture, keep hip bones facing forward as you gently turn to the right. Do not allow hips to turn (can cause stress to the knees).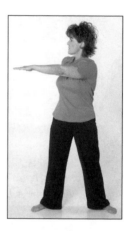

- Bring right hand to the back of right hip, gently pushing it forward.

- Bring left arm across your body to the right. Look to the right, breathing gently.

- Keep hips facing forward and reach out through your left hand.

- Exhale back to the center. Ponder the Scripture.

- Repeat on the left side.

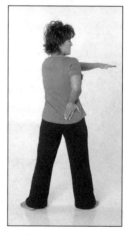

REST AND STRETCH

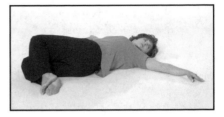

"Come to Me, all you who labor and are heavy laden, and I will give you rest" (Matthew 11:28).

Benefit: Promotes flexibility and strength in lower back and legs.

- While on your back, reach arms out to your sides, feet on the floor.
- Exhale, dropping your knees to the right, looking to the left.
- Hold for three to five breaths.
- Meditate on the Scripture.
- Inhale and then exhale, lifting knees. Repeat on the left side.

THE VINE

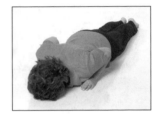

"I am the vine, you are the branches. He who abides in Me, and I in him, bears much fruit; for without Me you can do nothing" (John 15:5).

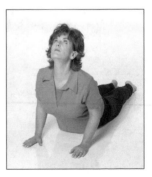

Benefit: Strengthens back and arms, stretches spine.

- Lie down on abdomen. Keep legs together, hands by your chest, elbows close to body.
- Inhaling, slowly raise head and chest as high as is comfortable. Keep glutes tight to protect lower back. Pelvis stays on floor.
- Repeat the Scripture out loud or to yourself. Breathe gently and deeply. Check your body to make sure you are not tensing up.

- Meditate on the Scripture.
- Hold the posture for three to five breaths. Relax and repeat.

THE LITTLE CHILD

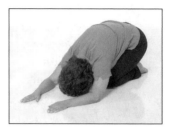

"Assuredly, I say to you, whoever does not receive the kingdom of God as a little child will by no means enter it" (Mark 10:15).

Benefit: Relaxes back and whole body. A good posture to do after any backward-bending floor posture.

- From abdomen, push off the floor with hands, facedown, rest on haunches.
- Arms in front or at sides, forehead or face down on mat.
- Relax, breathing gently for three to five deep breaths.
- Ponder the Scripture.
- Inhale and then exhale, pushing off your hands to come up.

DAVID'S HARP

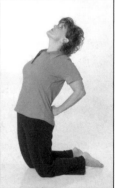

"Awake, lute and harp! I will awaken the dawn. I will praise You, O LORD, among the peoples, and I will sing praises to You among the nations" (Psalm 108:2-3).

Benefit: Strengthens legs and arms, stretches spine. Great for the lumbar region of lower back.

- *Beginner:* Kneeling, place fists toward back of hips and gently bow back, looking toward ceiling.
- Repeat the Scripture out loud or to yourself. Breathe gently and deeply. Check your body to make sure you are not tensing up.

- Meditate upon the Scripture.
- Hold the posture for three to five breaths. Relax.
- Exhale to release.
- Repeat Little Child pose to relax.
- *Advanced:* Kneeling, carefully reach back and grab your heels or ankles. Push hips forward, look up at ceiling.

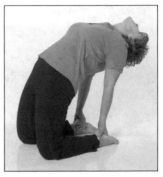

- Exhale and release both ankles at once, straightening up.
- Repeat Little Child pose to relax.

FLAPPING TENT

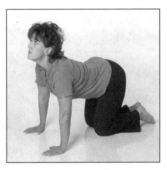

"The Spirit of God has made me, and the breath of the Almighty gives me life" (Job 33:4).

Benefit: Increases flexibility of the spine, works abdominal muscles.

- Start on hands and knees, keeping your hands just in front of your shoulders, legs about hip width apart.
- Inhale, tilting the tailbone up and let spine curve downward, dropping the abdomen and lifting your head up. Stretch gently.

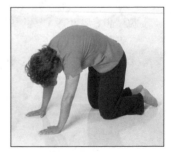

- Repeat the Scripture out loud or to yourself.
- Meditate on the Scripture.

- Exhale and reverse the spinal bend, tilting the tailbone down, pulling the chest and abdomen in.
- Gracefully flow from one to the other three or four times, reminiscent of the wind blowing in and out of a tent.

THE TENT

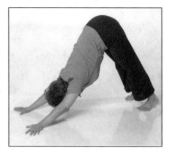

"Enlarge the place of your tent, and let them stretch out the curtains of your dwellings; do not spare; lengthen your cords, and strengthen your stakes" (Isaiah 54:2).

Benefit: Builds strength and flexibility, stretches spine and hamstrings.

- Begin on your hands and knees, legs hip width apart and arms shoulder width apart. Keep your middle fingers parallel, pointing straight ahead. Roll your elbows so that your inner elbows are facing forward.
- Inhale, arching your spine. Curl your toes under, as if getting ready to stand. As you exhale, straighten your legs and pause here for a moment.
- Exhale, pushing the floor away from your hands and straightening your legs, so your body looks like an inverted *V*. There should be a straight line from your hands through your shoulders to the hips.
- Press down on your hands between your index fingers and thumbs.
- Press your heels down toward the floor.
- Keep your arms and legs straight—like the lengthened cords and stakes of a tent.
- The goal of the Tent posture is to lengthen the spine while keeping your legs straight and feet flat on the ground. At

first, you may need to bend your knees slightly and keep your heels raised.

- Keep shoulders down and relaxed. Weight should be evenly distributed between hands and feet. Hold the position for a few breaths. Exhale as you release. Repeat several times. This is a challenging posture, so take it easy. You'll build up strength with practice.

- Repeat the Scripture before or after the posture until you know it well enough to say it while doing the Tent pose.

- Rest after this posture on your back with knees bent, or carefully walk hands to your feet, hanging as in the Tallit posture and then slowly rounding up, holding abdomen in all the way up to Mount Zion posture.

THE ALTAR

"I beseech you therefore, brethren, by the mercies of God, that you present your bodies a living sacrifice, holy, acceptable to God, which is your reasonable service" (Romans 12:1).

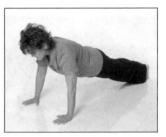

Benefit: Strengthens arms, upper back, and shoulders.

- On your hands and knees, bring your hands directly below your shoulders. Bring your knees together, toes curled under.

- Exhaling, straighten right leg, then left leg, keeping your weight balanced between your hands and toes.

- Lower your hips to form a straight line from your shoulders to your legs. Don't let your hips rise up.

- Hold the abdomen in.

- Relax and breathe gently.

- Ponder the Scripture.

- Release on the exhalation, bringing your knees down and coming back to all fours.

- Repeat several times.

WWJD Relaxation and Meditation Time

After practicing the PraiseMoves postures, relax on your back for a while. If your lower back is sensitive, bend your knees or put a pillow under them. Bring your arms to your sides, palms up. Relax your body from the top of your head to the soles of your feet. Make sure your neck and shoulders are not holding any tension.

Meditate on one or more of the Scriptures you focused on earlier. Fellowship with the Lord. If you have any cares, unconfessed sin, or unforgiveness, now is a good time to get rid of them. Rest in His presence and let Him love you.

Are you trusting God for healing? Now is a good time to receive your healing from the Lord, while you're completely relaxed in His presence.

More PraiseMoves

You have just experienced 15 of the basic PraiseMoves postures. Are your ready for more? Visit www.PraiseMoves.com for more information about…

PraiseMoves Alphabetics are 22 postures that mirror the Hebrew alphabet. These postures will help you meditate on Psalm 119. This is an acrostic psalm, meaning each verse begins with a different letter of the Hebrew alphabet from *aleph* through *tav* (we would say "*a* to *z*").

PraiseMoves Scripture Sequences are postures that flow gently from one to another while you say The Lord's Prayer, the Twenty-third Psalm, and other portions of Scripture. These graceful postures respectfully mirror the beauty of God's Word, allowing you to worship and meditate while you "glorify God in your body and in your spirit, which are God's."[9]

PraiseMoves teacher certification is now available. Depending on the source, 15 to 20 million people practice yoga in the United States, and 50,000 to 75,000 yoga instructors offer classes at an estimated 10,000 to 30,000 sites.[10] Imagine what an effective evangelistic tool "The Christian Alternative to Yoga" could be!

Bringing It Home

In this chapter I learned:

1. _____

2. _____

3. _____

I can start doing this better today: _____

_____

Lord, I ask You to help me _____

_____

10

*The Step-UP Program: 21 Days
to a Not-So-Extreme Makeover
by God's Design*

*For as the body without the spirit is dead,
so faith without works is dead also.*

JAMES 2:26

K NOWLEDGE IS VITAL, yet we can know everything there is to know about fitness and nutrition and still be out of shape and miserable. People can read books and listen to sermons by some of the most gifted Bible teachers and preachers of all time and still miss out on God's most precious gift—salvation—if all they do is listen and read. Success in any area of life requires action—not ignorant "fly by the seat of our pants" action but action coupled with knowledge and faith.

Since "faith is the substance of things hoped for," we need to know what we're hoping for! Hope is the blueprint your faith follows. Did you write down some personal goals and heartfelt prayers in chapter 8? If not, I strongly urge you to do so. Your faith needs a blueprint to follow. I invite you to write a brief blueprint for the Step-UP program below.

1. This is what I would like to accomplish during the next three weeks on the Step-UP program:

_____

_____

2. These are habits I'd like to develop and ones I want to overcome (spiritually, emotionally, mentally, and physically):

I want to stop_____

_____

And I want to start _____

_____

3. By continuing to follow the healthy guidelines of the Step-UP program as a lifestyle, one year from now I will have grown (spiritually, mentally, emotionally, physically) in these ways:

_____

_____

_____

The desires, plans, goals, and prayers you've just written down are your blueprint. These are your hopes. Hope is not a wishy-washy "wouldn't it be nice" idea. Hope is a spiritual *force*. In its purest biblical sense, *hope* means "earnest expectation." It carries with it the picture of a runner at top speed, pressing forward with intense determination as she heads for the finish line only a nose away. She earnestly expects to win. That's hope.

My *earnest expectation* is not only that *BASIC Steps* has given you head knowledge about fitness and health, but also that it has helped fuel your heart's desires to be all God has created you to be.

During the next three weeks you will put into practice many of the Body And Soul In Christ steps we've learned about in previous chapters. Behavioral science tells us we need at least 21 days to break an old habit and develop a new one. If you will commit to follow this program for three weeks, it can become the foundation of a new Christ-centered fitness lifestyle that will have a positive impact on you and your family. So Step-UP and praise the Lord as we move to higher levels of fitness in Him!

Step-UP Program Guidelines

1. Weigh and measure yourself and write the numbers down in your notebook. Do not weigh or measure again until after you have completed the program. Yes, I know that's difficult!

2. Sign the Step-UP Commitment later in this chapter. You may want to make a copy of it and keep it in your Bible or journal.

3. Write a BASIC food and exercise plan every day following the guidelines of the Food Circle and other suggestions (such as eating lots of veggies, limiting processed food). This will not be a diet but a food and exercise plan. I have found writing the following in my journal for each day helpful:

   Breakfast:

   Snack:

   Lunch:

   Snack:

   Dinner:

   Exercise:

Eating healthy foods every few hours fuels the body and enables it to burn fat more efficiently while keeping you energized. I commit my food for the day to the Lord and ask Him to guide me in making healthy choices. You can write out *exactly* what you are going to eat or an *outline* of what you will eat. An outline might look like this:

   Breakfast: fruit, carb

   Snack: fruit

   Lunch: protein, carb, salad, fat

   Snack: veggies

   Dinner: salad, protein, carb, fat

Carb represents foods such as whole grain bread, cereals, brown rice, and whole wheat pasta. *Protein* includes lean meat or soy, eggs, grains and beans, and dairy products. Avoid saturated *fats* and use other fats (such as butter and oil) sparingly. Take flaxseed oil or Omega 3 fish oil capsules daily for essential fatty acids. I take dietary supplements and vitamins daily, and I strongly recommend you do too. If you're not taking any vitamins, go to the health food store and ask for the best whole food multivitamin you can find (no cheapies— your body deserves the best). You can find my recommendations at www.BasicSteps.info.

Using an outline form of the Food Plan is often easier for people who eat out a lot. A more exact Food Plan may be difficult for some to follow (we don't want anyone falling apart because they "messed up"). Experiment to determine which works better for you. You will experience more success if you consider this a *lifestyle* plan—something you can easily live with that becomes second nature to you— more than a diet you can jump on or fall off.

BASIC Steps to Follow

1. Use a new journal or notebook to follow the three-week program.

2. Limit processed foods. That means even low-carb or low-fat processed foods. But don't be unrealistic about this, or you might quit. We can sometimes be "all or nothing" thinkers. Strive to eat foods as close to their natural state (as God made them) as possible. I was addicted to low-carb bars until I began limiting processed foods, and I'm now losing some of the "stubborn chub" that wouldn't let go. Your body processes veggies and fruit better than synthetic chemicals, preservatives, and natural or artificial flavors and colors.

3. Get adequate rest. Strive for seven to nine hours a night. Do the best you can—aim for progress, not perfection.

4. Practice a Tummy Curfew—stop eating three hours before bedtime.

5. Drink at least eight eight-ounce glasses of water daily. If you want to lose weight, divide your weight in half and drink that amount in ounces. For example, if you weigh 160 pounds,

drink eighty ounces—or ten eight-ounce glasses of water. If you drink no water at all, start with two to four glasses of water a day. Once you start limiting processed foods and eating more fruits and vegetables, you will find your natural thirst for water increasing.

6. Exercise 20 to 40 minutes each day. You might choose to take Sunday off—or just go for a lovely walk with the family. It's up to you. What kind of exercise? Any kind you will do! This includes the Gimme Ten Workout, walking on a treadmill or outdoors, rebounding (bouncing on a mini-trampoline), going to an exercise class, swimming, bicycling, jogging, doing a PraiseMoves or other exercise video...hey—if you're into roller blading or rock climbing, go for it!

   You can divide exercise into 10 to 15 minute segments if you want. If you're at the computer all day, take a break every few hours and walk around or do *something* that requires your body to *move*.

7. Spend time with the Lord every day. This is vital for spiritual fitness. Commit your day, your work, your food and exercise plan—everything concerning you—to the Lord first thing in the morning. Use a Bible translation you can easily understand, and follow along with our daily devotion. During the next three weeks you will read through the four Gospels with our primary emphasis on the words of Jesus. As much as possible, do your Bible reading in the morning. If you run short of time, finish the reading at bedtime. Do your best.

THE STEP-UP COMMITMENT

I, _____, hereby commit to improve my health and fitness for the next three weeks, beginning _____, 20__. I will eat healthful meals and snacks to nourish and energize my body, not to feed my emotions. I will make a conscious effort to move my body for 20 to 40 minutes six or seven days a week to improve my level of fitness and make exercise a part of my lifestyle.

In addition, during this period of time I will not indulge in eating the following foods I believe the Lord is guiding me to stop eating, regardless of the temptation:

_____

I will practice a Tummy Curfew and stop eating three hours before bedtime.

I purpose to spend time with the Lord every day and draw closer to Him. I am determined to know Him better than I ever have before, realizing that He is the source of everything good in my life. During this time, I believe He will change me more into the person He called me to be. I refuse to allow the past and self-defeating habits to keep me from being and doing all God wants me to be and do.

My body is the temple of the Holy Spirit, so I am learning to take better care of it.

This contract is with myself. I can also commit it to God if I so choose. Keeping this contract or breaking it is completely up to me. It carries with it no rewards or penalties other than those associated with its reflection on my ability to keep my word and the strength of my character.

I can do all things through Christ who strengthens me.

Signature: _____

Date: _____

Okay, that's it! I suggest you not "pig out" the day before you start! I know how I am, so I had to say that. Remember, even though you may be doing this only for a relatively short period of time, it's not a diet. This is about embracing a healthy lifestyle and drawing closer to the Lord, the One who makes all lasting change possible. I hope you'll continue to follow some of these guidelines in the future just because you enjoy the way you feel when you're doing them. You may choose to repeat the Step-UP program after three weeks, turning it into a six-week program if you'd like. It's up to you.

DAY ONE

Bible reading: Matthew, chapters 1 through 5

Scripture for today (write it in your journal): "But He answered and said, 'It is written, "Man shall not live by bread alone, but by every word that proceeds from the mouth of God."'" (Matthew 4:4).

What does it mean? Temptations will come whether we are starting a new fitness routine or just going about our daily lives. Since we are to follow Christ's example, let's do as Jesus did when faced with temptation: Answer back with the Word of God. Putting our fingers in our ears and saying, "No, no, no, devil!" will only go so far. Quoting God's Word as Jesus did puts the power of God to work in the situation. Find Scriptures that address your circumstances and regardless of what the physical circumstances may say, declare what *God* has to say about the situation! Physical food brings nourishment to the body, but only the Word of God can bring victory, fulfillment, and peace to your heart and soul.

Proclamation (say it aloud): I live and move and have my being in Christ, the Word of the living God. I choose to conform my words to His Word. I do not live by physical food alone but by every word that God has spoken to me in His Word. I praise You, Father, with my whole heart for who You are to me. *(Praise Him for who He is and all He's done.)*

What is the Lord saying to me in this Scripture? (Write it in your journal.)

Confession (start the day with a clean slate): Father, 1 John 1:9 says, "If we confess our sins, He is faithful and just to forgive us our sins and to cleanse us from all unrighteousness." I confess to You, repent and ask You to forgive me for these sins...*(say them to the Lord).*

Thank you for forgiving me, Lord. I now receive Your cleansing from all unrighteousness—from anything that stands between You and me—in Jesus' name. By Your grace I now stand clear and clean in Your sight. Thank You, Father!

Forgiveness (start the day with a clean heart): Father, Jesus said in Mark 11:25, "And whenever you stand praying, if you have anything against anyone, forgive him, that your Father in heaven may also forgive you your trespasses." Father, as You have forgiven me, and in obedience to Your Word, I forgive and let go of these people *(in your journal, write the names of people you forgive).*

Requests: I pray for the leaders of our nation and those in authority.[1] I pray for the peace of Jerusalem[2] and for the safety and effectiveness of our military at home and overseas. I now lift up the needs of my family and friends *(write your requests for others in your journal).*

I offer up my personal prayers today. Lord, I pray for Your help and guidance *(write your personal requests in your journal).*

Jesus said, "Whatever things you ask when you pray, believe that you receive them, and you will have them."[3] I believe I receive the answer to my prayers now. Thank You, Father!

Food plan for today (breakfast, snack, lunch, snack, dinner. Write it in your journal).

Tummy curfew: I commit to stop eating three hours before bedtime.

Exercise plan for today (write it in your journal).

Top three goals for this year (write them in your journal).

Three things I commit to do today (write them in your journal).

I commit my day to the Lord. Lord, I entrust my day and my life to You. Thank You helping me start the Step-UP program. Help me to keep on track and guide me to be the best I can be today. I purpose to fill my mouth with Your words, Lord. I'll walk by faith, not by sight!

Reflections on the day (write tonight or tomorrow morning in your journal).

DAY TWO

Bible reading: Matthew, chapters 6 through 10

Scripture for today (write it in your journal): Jesus said, "But seek first the kingdom of God and His righteousness, and all these things shall be added to you" (Matthew 6:33).

What does it mean? "The kingdom of God" refers to God's way of doing things. An example of God's way of doing things can be found in the law of sowing and reaping. Whatever seeds we sow, whether for good or evil, will grow up according to their kind. If you plant tomato seeds, you get tomatoes. Plant years of inactivity and Twinkies, and you get a flabby body. The good news is that once we begin planting good seeds, we will eventually reap a good harvest—if we don't give up. You're planting good seeds by choosing to follow your program today.

How do we seek God's way of doing things? Reading and studying His Word, praying, and taking action on what God's Word says are some of the ways we do that. Instead of worrying about what we are to eat or wear or how a bill will be paid, look to God's way. For example, we give (or sow) before we receive (or harvest). You will most likely take a step of faith first and stand in faith, believing God's Word is true, before you actually see the physical manifestation of your answered prayers. Remember, "the just shall live by faith."[4]

Proclamation (say aloud): I seek first the kingdom of God—God's way of doing things. I thank You, Lord, that because You gave Your Son Jesus to redeem mankind, I am made righteous in Him.[5] I seek You, Lord, and I am grateful that You reward those who diligently seek You.[6] By faith I have everything I need. *(Praise Him for who He is and for meeting your every need.)*

What is the Lord saying to me in this Scripture? (Write it in your journal.)

Confession (start the day with a clean slate. Confess your sins, repent, and ask for God's forgiveness.)

Forgiveness (start the day with a clean heart. In your journal, write the names of people you forgive.)

Requests: I pray for the leaders of our nation and those in authority. I pray for the peace of Jerusalem and for the safety and effectiveness of our military at home and overseas. I now lift up the needs of my family and friends *(write your requests for others in your journal).*

I offer up my personal prayers today. Lord, I pray for Your help and guidance in these areas *(write your personal requests in your journal).*

Jesus said, "Whatever things you ask when you pray, believe that you receive them, and you will have them." I believe I receive the answer to my prayers now. Thank You, Father!

Food plan for today (*breakfast, snack, lunch, snack, dinner. Write it in your journal*).

Tummy curfew: I commit to stop eating three hours before bed-time.

Exercise plan for today (*write it in your journal*).

Top three goals for this year (*write them in your journal*).

Three things I commit to do today (*write them in your journal*).

I commit my day to the Lord. Lord, as I commit my day and plans to You, I thank You that I'm open to any change of plans You have for me. I'm Your child, and I seek to do Your will all day, every day. I love You, Father. I'm grateful I hear Your voice in my heart, and I follow You in Jesus' name. Amen.

Reflections on the day (*write tonight or tomorrow morning in your journal*).

DAY THREE

Bible reading: Matthew, chapters 11 through 14

Scripture for today (*write it in your journal*): "Either make the tree good and its fruit good, or make the tree bad and its fruit bad; for a tree is known by its fruit" (Matthew 12:33).

What does it mean? Just like an apple tree will yield fruit after its kind, the Spirit of God is yielding fruit in our lives after the Spirit. The nine fruit of the Spirit listed in Galatians 5:22 are love, joy, peace, patience, kindness, goodness, faithfulness, gentleness, and self-control. Every time we put to death the desires of the flesh to lash out in anger, give in to temptation, or follow any number of selfish "me first" desires, we are yielding to the fruit of the Spirit. The more we yield to the Spirit of God day by day, the stronger and healthier the good fruit becomes and the more we are transformed into the image of our Lord from glory to glory.[7]

Proclamation (*say aloud*): I thank You, Lord, that You are culti-vating the fruit of the Spirit in my life. I choose to yield to love, joy, peace, patience, kindness, goodness, faithfulness, gentleness, and self-control. (*Praise Him for who He is and for developing the fruit of the Spirit in your life.*)

What is the Lord saying to me in this Scripture? (*Write it in your journal.*)

Confession (*start the day with a clean slate. Confess your sins, repent, and ask for God's forgiveness.*)

Forgiveness (*start the day with a clean heart. In your journal, write the names of people you forgive.*)

Requests: I pray for the leaders of our nation and those in authority. I pray for the peace of Jerusalem and for the safety and effectiveness of our military at home and overseas. I now lift up the needs of my family and friends (*write your requests for others in your journal*).

I offer up my personal prayers today. Lord, I pray for Your help and guidance in these areas (*write your personal requests in your journal*).

Jesus said, "Whatever things you ask when you pray, believe that you receive them, and you will have them." I believe I receive the answer to my prayers now. Thank You, Father!

Food plan for today (*breakfast, snack, lunch, snack, dinner. Write it in your journal*).

Tummy curfew: I commit to stop eating three hours before bedtime.

Exercise plan for today (*write it in your journal*).

Top three goals for this year (*write them in your journal*).

Three things I commit to do today (*write them in your journal*).

I commit my day to the Lord. Lord, as I go about my day today, if I become tempted to yield to the bad fruit (the works of the flesh), I ask that You remind me to yield to the good fruit of the Spirit within me. I commit my day and my life to You today, and I ask You to help me be a blessing to all I meet.

Reflections on the day (*write tonight or tomorrow morning in your journal*).

DAY FOUR

Bible reading: Matthew, chapters 15 through 18

Scripture for today (*write it in your journal*): "Hear and understand: Not what goes into the mouth defiles a man; but what comes out of the mouth, this defiles a man" (Matthew 15:10-11).

What does it mean? Aren't you glad God isn't keeping information from us? He wants us to understand. His words to us are mysteries to be revealed rather than secrets that are concealed. Jesus said, "Hear and understand" because He wants us to comprehend and benefit from His words to us.

Unclean food may contaminate the body, but it cannot contaminate the spirit and soul as can the hateful, destructive words we speak.

Whatever our heart is full of will come out of our mouth. "A good man out of the good treasure of his heart brings forth good; and an evil man out of the evil treasure of his heart brings forth evil. For out of the abundance of the heart his mouth speaks" (Luke 6:45).

A country preacher once said, "When your bucket gets bumped, whatever you're full of will spill out." When your "bucket gets bumped," what are some of the words and emotions that spill out of you? Well, grab hold of your tongue and zip your lip if you have to! You don't have to say *everything* that comes to mind, you know (that was a revelation to me!).

As important as clean, healthy food is, make sure your *words* are equally unsoiled, positive, and full of the "nutrition" of God's Word.

Proclamation *(say aloud):* I will speak words of love, encouragement, and peace. God gives me wisdom to speak His Word even in the most trying of circumstances. When I open my mouth in faith, He gives me the perfect words to say. I will now praise Him with the sweet, clear words of my mouth. *(Praise Him for who He is and for filling your mouth with words of life.)*

What is the Lord saying to me in this Scripture? *(Write it in your journal.)*

Confession *(start the day with a clean slate. Confess your sins, repent, and ask for God's forgiveness.)*

Forgiveness *(start the day with a clean heart. In your journal, write the names of people you forgive.)*

Requests: I pray for the leaders of our nation and those in authority. I pray for the peace of Jerusalem and for the safety and effectiveness of our military at home and overseas. I now lift up the needs of my family and friends *(write your requests for others in your journal).*

I offer up my personal prayers today. Lord, I pray for Your help and guidance in these areas *(write your personal requests in your journal).*

Jesus said, "Whatever things you ask when you pray, believe that you receive them, and you will have them." I believe I receive the answer to my prayers now. Thank You, Father!

Food plan for today *(breakfast, snack, lunch, snack, dinner. Write it in your journal).*

Tummy curfew: I commit to stop eating three hours before bed-time.

Exercise plan for today *(write it in your journal).*

Top three goals for this year *(write them in your journal).*

Three things I commit to do today *(write them in your journal).*

I commit my day to the Lord. Lord, please keep a guard on my lips so I will not sin against You with my mouth. Please caution me in my heart if I am about to lie, gossip, or speak ill of someone. I say with David, "Let the words of my mouth and the meditation of my heart be acceptable in Your sight, O LORD, my strength and my Redeemer."[8]

Reflections on the day *(write tonight or tomorrow morning in your journal).*

DAY FIVE

Bible reading: Matthew, chapters 19 through 23

Scripture for today *(write it in your journal):* "So Jesus stood still and called them, and said, 'What do you want Me to do for you?'" (Matthew 20:32).

What does it mean? Why did Jesus ask those two blind men what they wanted Him to do for them? Surely He knew they were blind. Well, the Lord is not a puppet master. Instead of "pulling our strings," He wants us to tell Him what we want. Our words are also indicators of our faith. Obviously these men had faith that Jesus could heal them, for they answered Him, "Lord, that our eyes may be opened." And they were healed.

On several occasions in Scripture, when people were healed, the Lord told them, "Your *faith* has made you well (completely whole)."[9] However, in His hometown of Nazareth, "He could do no mighty work." In fact, "He marveled because of their unbelief."[10] Their sight was more limited than the blind men's. They refused to see beyond what they knew in the natural about Jesus: that He was a carpenter, the Son of Mary, and the brother of James, Joses, Judas, and Simon. Their lack of faith in Him kept them from receiving anything from God.

Jesus is asking you today, "What do you want Me to do for you?" Be specific, put your faith in Him, and you too will be made completely whole.

Proclamation (say aloud): I will be specific in what I ask the Lord to do for me. I am not afraid to ask Him because I know He wants to be involved in every area of my life. Jesus, I will answer Your question, "What do you want Me to do for you?" I come boldly to the throne of grace that I may obtain mercy and find grace to help in the time of need.[11] Lord I ask You... *(ask the Lord to help you in the specific areas you want His help. Praise Him for who He is and for answering your prayers.)*

What is the Lord saying to me in this Scripture? *(Write it in your journal.)*

Confession *(start the day with a clean slate. Confess your sins, repent, and ask for God's forgiveness.)*

Forgiveness *(start the day with a clean heart. In your journal, write the names of people you forgive.)*

Requests: I pray for the leaders of our nation and those in authority. I pray for the peace of Jerusalem and for the safety and effectiveness of our military at home and overseas. I now lift up the needs of my family and friends *(write your requests for others in your journal).*

I offer up my personal prayers today. Lord, I pray for Your help and guidance in these areas *(write your personal requests in your journal).*

Jesus said, "Whatever things you ask when you pray, believe that you receive them, and you will have them." I believe I receive the answer to my prayers now. Thank You, Father!

Food plan for today *(breakfast, snack, lunch, snack, dinner. Write it in your journal).*

Tummy curfew: I commit to stop eating three hours before bedtime.

Exercise plan for today *(write it in your journal).*

Top three goals for this year *(write them in your journal).*

Three things I commit to do today *(write them in your journal).*

I commit my day to the Lord. Lord, I entrust my day and my life to You. I put everything in Your hands today. Thank You for always being with me and for answering my prayers. I'm so grateful to be Your child, knowing I can come to You at any time and receive Your help, wisdom, and love.

Reflections on the day *(write tonight or tomorrow morning in your journal).*

DAY SIX

Bible reading: Matthew, chapters 24 through 26

Scripture for today (write it in your journal): "Watch and pray, lest you enter into temptation. The spirit indeed is willing, but the flesh is weak" (Matthew 26:41).

What does it mean? The more time we spend in the things of God, the stronger and more sensitive our spirit becomes, enabling us to overcome the temptations of the flesh. The word for "watch" in the Greek is *gregoreuo*, meaning to refrain from sleep or be watchful and awake mentally and spiritually.

Be mindful of the thoughts you are entertaining. Are they of God, the flesh, or the devil? If they are not of God, cast them down (kick them out!) and bring "every thought into captivity to the obedience of Christ."[12]

Many are lulled to sleep and unaware of the snares of the enemy until after they've been caught. Peter tells us to "be sober [self-controlled], be vigilant [watchful]; because your adversary the devil walks about like a roaring lion, seeking whom he may devour" (1 Peter 5:8).

Enjoying frequent fellowship with God and taking action on what you know to do will strengthen your spirit and cultivate the fruits of faithfulness, patient endurance, and self-control.

Proclamation (say aloud): With Paul I can say that I am not ignorant of the devil's devices.[13] I will spend time in prayer and fellowship with the Lord every day. Under the leadership of the Lord Jesus Christ, my spirit is in control over my flesh. When tempted, I will not enter in but will immediately go to Jesus in the Word and in prayer. I am an overcomer and am being "strengthened with might through His Spirit in the inner man"[14] (in my spirit). *(Praise the Lord for who He is and for strengthening your spirit.)*

What is the Lord saying to me in this Scripture? (Write it in your journal.)

Confession (start the day with a clean slate. Confess your sins, repent, and ask for God's forgiveness.)

Forgiveness (start the day with a clean heart. In your journal, write the names of people you forgive.)

Requests: I pray for the leaders of our nation and those in authority. I pray for the peace of Jerusalem and for the safety and effectiveness of our military at home and overseas. I now lift up the needs of my family and friends *(write your requests for others in your journal).*

I offer up my personal prayers today. Lord, I pray for Your help and guidance in these areas *(write your personal requests in your journal).*

Jesus said, "Whatever things you ask when you pray, believe that you receive them, and you will have them." I believe I receive the answer to my prayers now. Thank You, Father!

Food plan for today *(breakfast, snack, lunch, snack, dinner. Write it in your journal).*

Tummy curfew: I commit to stop eating three hours before bedtime.

Exercise plan for today *(write it in your journal).*

Top three goals for this year *(write them in your journal).*

Three things I commit to do today *(write them in your journal).*

I commit my day to the Lord. Lord, thank You for strengthening me in my spirit, soul, and body today. I will be watchful today and sensitive to do what Your Holy Spirit tells me. I place my day, my life, and my plans completely in Your hands, Lord, and I thank You for Your great, great love for me and my family!

Reflections on the day *(write tonight or tomorrow morning in your journal).*

DAY SEVEN

Bible reading: Matthew 27 through Mark 3

Scripture for today *(write it in your journal):* "A leper came…saying to Him, 'If You are willing, You can make me clean.' Then Jesus, moved with compassion, stretched out His hand and touched him, and said to him, 'I am willing; be cleansed'" (Mark 1:40-41).

What does it mean? We are told in Hebrews 13:8 that "Jesus Christ is the same yesterday, today, and forever." If He was willing to touch an outcast with compassion and healing 2000 years ago, He is still willing today. Jesus specialized in doing the impossible—because with God *nothing* is impossible! He is still willing to save, heal, and deliver all who ask in faith.

If you wonder whether your faith is strong enough, realize God has already given you the faith that you need. The faith you have can be strengthened by reading, speaking, and hearing the Word of God.

So, take action on the Word of God that you know, and your faith "muscles" will grow!

Jesus is moved with compassion toward us and through us to others. Notice that He stretched out His hand to touch the leper *before* He said anything. We are His hands here on earth. Even if we don't know what to say to someone who's hurting, we can stretch out our hand to them, and the Lord will give us the words to say.

God desires to touch you with His love, grace, and power right now. Whatever you have been asking the Lord about or standing in faith believing, realize that His hand is stretched out to touch you right now. He is speaking to you today: "I am willing; be cleansed."

Proclamation *(say aloud):* I praise the Lord that He is willing and able to perform His Word in my life. I humble myself under the mighty outstretched hand of God, that He may exalt me in due time. I cast all my care upon Him, for He cares for me.[15] *(Praise the Lord for who He is and for bringing to pass His promises in your life.)*

What is the Lord saying to me in this Scripture? *(Write it in your journal.)*

Confession *(start the day with a clean slate. Confess your sins, repent, and ask for God's forgiveness.)*

Forgiveness *(start the day with a clean heart. In your journal, write the names of people you forgive.)*

Requests: I pray for the leaders of our nation and those in authority. I pray for the peace of Jerusalem and for the safety and effectiveness of our military at home and overseas. I now lift up the needs of my family and friends *(write your requests for others in your journal).*

I offer up my personal prayers today. Lord, I pray for Your help and guidance in these areas *(write your personal requests in your journal).*

Jesus said, "Whatever things you ask when you pray, believe that you receive them, and you will have them." I believe I receive the answer to my prayers now. Thank You, Father!

Food plan for today *(breakfast, snack, lunch, snack, dinner. Write it in your journal).*

Tummy curfew: I commit to stop eating three hours before bedtime.

Exercise plan for today *(write it in your journal).*

Top three goals for this year *(write them in your journal).*

Three things I commit to do today *(write them in your journal).*

I commit my day to the Lord. Lord, I commit my day and my life to You. I thank You that You are willing and able to watch over everything I entrust to You. I am so grateful my life is in Your hands.

Reflections on the day (write tonight or tomorrow morning in your journal).

DAY EIGHT

Bible reading: Mark, chapters 4 through 7

Scripture for today (write it in your journal): "Daughter, your faith has made you well. Go in peace, and be healed of your affliction" (Mark 5:34).

What does it mean? Here we meet a woman who had experienced pain and misery for years. She was weakened physically from her condition and had suffered from the treatments of the physicians as well. For 12 long years her illness made her unclean under Jewish law, so she was ostracized from society. She had also spent all her money trying to regain her health.

How did she receive her healing? (1) She heard about Jesus and believed. (2) She spoke her faith aloud to herself: "If only I may touch His clothes, I shall be made well." (3) She took action. She touched His clothes in faith, believing she would get what she needed from Him. (4) She received her healing from Jesus by faith.

Her faith obviously drew on the power of the Lord. "And Jesus, immediately knowing in Himself that *power had gone out of Him,* turned around in the crowd and said, 'Who touched My clothes?'" Many people touched Jesus that day, but one touched Him in faith. That woman's faith was the bridge that brought the power to heal from Jesus to her. It wasn't her need that drew the power, but her faith.

You can follow those same four steps today. (1) Find a promise in the Word of God to fit your situation. (2) Speak God's promise aloud and claim it for yourself. (3) Take action. Push past the obstacles standing between you and Jesus, between you and your healing, between you and the answer to your prayer. (4) Receive it. Believe right now that you are receiving the answer to your prayer. Then thank the Lord with your whole heart. There's power in praising Him!

Proclamation (say aloud): Lord, I hear Your Word and believe it. I speak it out loud in faith. I take action on Your Word and push past all obstacles standing in my way. I receive Your wonderful promises by faith and walk in victory! *(Praise the Lord for who He is and for making His power available to you today.)*

What is the Lord saying to me in this Scripture? *(Write it in your journal.)*

Confession *(start the day with a clean slate. Confess your sins, repent, and ask for God's forgiveness.)*

Forgiveness *(start the day with a clean heart. In your journal, write the names of people you forgive.)*

Requests: I pray for the leaders of our nation and those in authority. I pray for the peace of Jerusalem and for the safety and effectiveness of our military at home and overseas. I now lift up the needs of my family and friends *(write your requests for others in your journal).*

I offer up my personal prayers today. Lord, I pray for Your help and guidance in these areas *(write your personal requests in your journal).*

Jesus said, "Whatever things you ask when you pray, believe that you receive them, and you will have them." I believe I receive the answer to my prayers now. Thank You, Father!

Food plan for today *(breakfast, snack, lunch, snack, dinner. Write it in your journal).*

Tummy curfew: I commit to stop eating three hours before bedtime.

Exercise plan for today *(write it in your journal).*

Top three goals for this year *(write them in your journal).*

Three things I commit to do today *(write them in your journal).*

I commit my day to the Lord. Lord, I refuse to allow anything to stand between us. I am a child of the King, and I'm pressing in to be all He's called me to be.

Reflections on the day *(write tonight or tomorrow morning in your journal).*

DAY NINE

Bible reading: Mark, chapters 8 through 11

Scripture for today *(write it in your journal):* "Assuredly, I say to you, whoever does not receive the kingdom of God as a little child will by no means enter it" (Mark 10:15).

What does it mean? If the kingdom of God refers to God's way of doing things, and we must receive and understand it as a little child would, we run the risk of missing out on much of what the Lord has for us by being too "grown-up."

Grown-ups say, "I'll believe it when I see it." Children say, "I believe it, so I know I'm going to see it!" Grown-ups say, "Don't get your hopes up." Children say, "Too late. My hopes are way up!" Bible-based faith is similarly childlike, but it's not childish.

Faith is the currency, the "coin of the realm," of the kingdom of God. Faith is believing and acting with the calm assurance that the Word of God is true—no matter what the circumstances may say. Circumstances are only temporary; God's Word is eternal.

Are you facing a situation that seems impossible? How would a Bible-believing child view that situation? Today you read about Jesus telling His disciples, "With men it is impossible, but not with God; for with God all things are possible."[16]

Receive God's way of doing things like a child today. Don't hoard your faith—spend it! Pour your faith into something huge, gigantic, and stupendous (just like a child would!). God turns the impossible into the possible, and the possible into reality!

Proclamation *(say aloud):* Lord, I know that with You all things are possible. I stretch my faith out like a child today and thank You in advance for turning impossible situations around. Thank You for making a way where there seemed to be no way. I am excited about what You are doing in my life and the lives of my loved ones. *(Praise the Lord for who He is and for restoring your childlike faith.)*

What is the Lord saying to me in this Scripture? *(Write it in your journal.)*

Confession *(start the day with a clean slate. Confess your sins, repent, and ask for God's forgiveness.)*

Forgiveness *(start the day with a clean heart. In your journal, write the names of people you forgive.)*

Requests: I pray for the leaders of our nation and those in authority. I pray for the peace of Jerusalem and for the safety and effectiveness of our military at home and overseas. I now lift up the needs of my family and friends *(write your requests for others in your journal).*

I offer up my personal prayers today. Lord, I pray for Your help and guidance in these areas *(write your personal requests in your journal).*

Jesus said, "Whatever things you ask when you pray, believe that you receive them, and you will have them." I believe I receive the answer to my prayers now. Thank You, Father!

Food plan for today *(breakfast, snack, lunch, snack, dinner. Write it in your journal).*

Tummy curfew: I commit to stop eating three hours before bedtime.

Exercise plan for today *(write it in your journal).*

Top three goals for this year *(write them in your journal).*

Three things I commit to do today *(write them in your journal).*

I commit my day to the Lord. Lord, I receive the kingdom of God as a little child, and I enter it by faith. Thank You for showing me how to operate as an ambassador of this kingdom, as an ambassador of Christ. Please give me the words to say to encourage others to trust You like a child and walk before You like men and women of God.

Reflections on the day *(write tonight or tomorrow morning in your journal).*

DAY TEN

Bible reading: Mark, chapters 12 through 14

Scripture for today *(write it in your journal):* " 'You shall love the LORD your God with all your heart, with all your soul, with all your mind, and with all your strength.' This is the first commandment. And the second, like it, is this: 'You shall love your neighbor as yourself.' There is no other commandment greater than these" (Mark 12:30-31).

What does it mean? We miss a lot if we just glance over these Scriptures thinking God gave us these commandments just because He didn't want us to be drawn away into idol worship. Everything God does is for our benefit and out of His enormous love for us.

While pondering this Scripture, I saw how immensely practical the Lord is. By making the primary commandment love, God is helping us to grow several different ways. (1) He is enabling us to stay close to Him ("God is love"[17]). (2) He is teaching us to give sacrificially ("For God so *loved* the world that He *gave* His only begotten Son"[18]). (3) He is helping us build our faith ("faith working through love"[19]).

(4) He is giving us a weapon to fight fear ("Perfect love casts out fear"[20]). (5) He is ensuring our victory ("Love never fails"[21]).

Let's identify with love today by inserting ourselves into 1 Corinthians 13:4-8 with the following:

Proclamation *(say aloud):* By God's grace I identify with the love of God. I will be patient and kind. I will not envy. I will not parade myself or show off, nor will I be puffed up with pride. I will not behave rudely, nor will I seek after my own fulfillment or gratification. I will not be easily provoked. I will think no evil. I will not rejoice in evil, but I will rejoice in the truth. I will bear all things, believe all things, hope all things, and endure all things. I will never fail because love never fails. Love never fails because God never fails, and God is love. *(Praise the Lord for who He is and for filling you with His love.)*

What is the Lord saying to me in this Scripture? *(Write it in your journal.)*

Confession *(start the day with a clean slate. Confess your sins, repent, and ask for God's forgiveness.)*

Forgiveness *(start the day with a clean heart. In your journal, write the names of people you forgive.)*

Requests: I pray for the leaders of our nation and those in authority. I pray for the peace of Jerusalem and for the safety and effectiveness of our military at home and overseas. I now lift up the needs of my family and friends *(write your requests for others in your journal).*

I offer up my personal prayers today. Lord, I pray for Your help and guidance in these areas *(write your personal requests in your journal).*

Jesus said, "Whatever things you ask when you pray, believe that you receive them, and you will have them." I believe I receive the answer to my prayers now. Thank You, Father!

Food plan for today *(breakfast, snack, lunch, snack, dinner. Write it in your journal).*

Tummy curfew: I commit to stop eating three hours before bedtime.

Exercise plan for today *(write it in your journal).*

Top three goals for this year *(write them in your journal).*

Three things I commit to do today *(write them in your journal).*

I commit my day to the Lord. Lord, I love You with all my heart and soul, and with all the wealth and resources I possess. I hold nothing back from You. I love my neighbor as I love myself. I am able to love,

Lord, because You first loved me. I do not hate myself, nor do I hate others. I choose to walk in love today, and I will not fulfill the selfish desires of my carnal nature.

Reflections on the day (write tonight or tomorrow morning in your journal).

DAY ELEVEN

Bible reading: Mark 15 through Luke 2

Scripture for today (write it in your journal): "Behold the maidservant of the Lord! Let it be to me according to your word" (Luke 1:38).

What does it mean? Mary didn't understand everything that would happen when the angel Gabriel told her she would give birth to the Son of God. She could not have comprehended the magnitude of what God was about to do on earth. Still, she showed her willingness to trust and obey the Lord, calling herself His maidservant.

The prophet Isaiah offered a similar exclamation when He heard the voice of the Lord saying, "Whom shall I send, and who will go for Us?" (Isaiah 6:8). Even though Isaiah considered himself less than worthy and "a man of unclean lips," he said, "Here am I! Send me." Notice that God did not hesitate. When He found a willing vessel, He immediately said, "Go!"

God is calling you to be His maidservant and a vessel of His power today. Is this because you are worthy of such an honor? No, but He is. A great woman of God once said, "God is not looking for vessels of gold or silver but for *yielded* vessels."

Proclamation (say aloud): I will go where God wants me to go, do what God wants me to do, and say what God wants me to say today. With Mary I proclaim, "Behold the maidservant of the Lord! Let it be to me according to Your word." And with Isaiah I say, "Here am I! Send me." God said He would never leave me nor forsake me, so I know He goes with me, gives me favor with those I meet, and He will give me the words to say. *(Praise the Lord for who He is and for the calling He has placed on your life.)*

What is the Lord saying to me in this Scripture? (Write it in your journal.)

Confession *(start the day with a clean slate. Confess your sins, repent, and ask for God's forgiveness.)*

Forgiveness *(start the day with a clean heart. In your journal, write the names of people you forgive.)*

Requests: I pray for the leaders of our nation and those in authority. I pray for the peace of Jerusalem and for the safety and effectiveness of our military at home and overseas. I now lift up the needs of my family and friends *(write your requests for others in your journal).*

I offer up my personal prayers today. Lord, I pray for Your help and guidance in these areas *(write your personal requests in your journal).*

Jesus said, "Whatever things you ask when you pray, believe that you receive them, and you will have them." I believe I receive the answer to my prayers now. Thank You, Father!

Food plan for today *(breakfast, snack, lunch, snack, dinner. Write it in your journal).*

Tummy curfew: I commit to stop eating three hours before bedtime.

Exercise plan for today *(write it in your journal).*

Top three goals for this year *(write them in your journal).*

Three things I commit to do today *(write them in your journal).*

I commit my day to the Lord. Lord, I pray Your will be done on earth today as it is in heaven. Thank You for sending me into my world to make a difference. Let it be to me according to Your Word, in Jesus' name.

Reflections on the day *(write tonight or tomorrow morning in your journal).*

DAY TWELVE

Bible reading: Luke, chapters 3 through 6

Scripture for today *(write it in your journal):* "Launch out into the deep and let down your nets for a catch" (Luke 5:4).

What does it mean? The Lord invites us to come to Him and receive everything we need, and we sheepishly hold out a thimble to carry home our blessings. Perhaps our poor self-image keeps us from receiving what the Lord has for us. Or maybe we don't really *expect* to receive much. What do you expect to receive from God?

Jesus told Peter to trust Him—to launch out into the deep water and let down his nets. Peter, an experienced fisherman, knew he had worked all night and caught nothing. His mind and circumstances said he would catch no fish that day, but to appease the Teacher, he agreed to let down one net. I doubt he even launched out very far from where they were. As you know, he caught so many fish that his net broke, and the crew filled two boats to the point of sinking. What would have happened if Peter had launched out into the deep and let down *all* their nets?

Is the Lord asking you to trust Him? Is He asking you to launch out into the deep and let down your "nets" for a haul? What is keeping you from taking action? Are you, like Peter, looking at the seeming impossibility of the situation you face? The supernatural is God's responsibility. At the word of the Lord, let down your nets for a huge, boat-sinking catch. He will fill it!

Proclamation *(say aloud):* I launch out into the deep and embrace all the Lord has for me today. I expect great things of my God and King. I am not conformed to this world, but I am being transformed by the renewing of my mind. By God's grace I am proving that good and acceptable and perfect will of God. *(Praise the Lord for who He is and for filling your "nets"!)*

What is the Lord saying to me in this Scripture? *(Write it in your journal.)*

Confession *(start the day with a clean slate. Confess your sins, repent, and ask for God's forgiveness.)*

Forgiveness *(start the day with a clean heart. In your journal, write the names of people you forgive.)*

Requests: I pray for the leaders of our nation and those in authority. I pray for the peace of Jerusalem and for the safety and effectiveness of our military at home and overseas. I now lift up the needs of my family and friends *(write your requests for others in your journal).*

I offer up my personal prayers today. Lord, I pray for Your help and guidance in these areas *(write your personal requests in your journal).*

Jesus said, "Whatever things you ask when you pray, believe that you receive them, and you will have them." I believe I receive the answer to my prayers now. Thank You, Father!

Food plan for today *(breakfast, snack, lunch, snack, dinner. Write it in your journal).*

Tummy curfew: I commit to stop eating three hours before bedtime.

Exercise plan for today (*write it in your journal*).

Top three goals for this year (*write them in your journal*).

Three things I commit to do today (*write them in your journal*).

I commit my day to the Lord. Lord, with You all things are possible, so I'm not afraid to launch out into the deep. When You tell me to take a step of faith and trust You today, I'll do it. No more thimblefuls for me! My nets are clean, mended, and ready for boatloads of Your grace, truth, and love. I receive them by faith and step forward with boldness today!

Reflections on the day (*write tonight or tomorrow morning in your journal*).

DAY THIRTEEN

Bible reading: Luke, chapters 7 through 9

Scripture for today (*write it in your journal*): "No one, having put his hand to the plow, and looking back, is fit for the kingdom of God" (Luke 9:62).

What does it mean? I've never physically put my hand to a plow to till the soil, but I've put my hand to a number of projects over the years. One of the main objectives when using a plow is to go forward in a straight line. If a farmer continues to look back over his shoulder at what he has already plowed, he'll start veering off in the wrong direction. I've made that mistake while driving, only to catch myself going off onto the shoulder of the road and correcting myself with a quick "Thank You, Jesus!"

The Amplified Bible offers greater clarity to Jesus' admonition, "No one who puts his hand to the plow and looks back [to the things behind] is fit for the kingdom of God." If the kingdom of God refers to God's way of doing things here and now, we know He doesn't want us to be imprisoned by the things of the past. Faith is walking a straight path forward regardless of what happened to discourage us ten years ago or ten *minutes* ago.

Perhaps you've looked back with longing to the way your life was when your children were small or when you were first married, to a long-lost love, or to the way your body looked when you were 18!

The Lord is telling us that dwelling on the past makes us unfit to operate in the kingdom of God today. It's not that He judges us unworthy but that we are unable to act in faith today if we are pausing to consider yesterday. Remember Lot's wife![22]

Proclamation *(say aloud):* I don't look back, but I look straight ahead. God is my source of all good. He is able to make all grace abound toward me, that I, always having all sufficiency in all things, may have an abundance for every good work.[23] *(Praise the Lord for who He is and for setting His joyous purpose before you.)*

What is the Lord saying to me in this Scripture? *(Write it in your journal.)*

Confession *(start the day with a clean slate. Confess your sins, repent, and ask for God's forgiveness.)*

Forgiveness *(start the day with a clean heart. In your journal, write the names of people you forgive.)*

Requests: I pray for the leaders of our nation and those in authority. I pray for the peace of Jerusalem and for the safety and effectiveness of our military at home and overseas. I now lift up the needs of my family and friends *(write your requests for others in your journal).*

I offer up my personal prayers today. Lord, I pray for Your help and guidance in these areas *(write your personal requests in your journal).*

Jesus said, "Whatever things you ask when you pray, believe that you receive them, and you will have them." I believe I receive the answer to my prayers now. Thank You, Father!

Food plan for today *(breakfast, snack, lunch, snack, dinner. Write it in your journal).*

Tummy curfew: I commit to stop eating three hours before bedtime.

Exercise plan for today *(write it in your journal).*

Top three goals for this year *(write them in your journal).*

Three things I commit to do today *(write them in your journal).*

I commit my day to the Lord. I entrust my day to You, Lord. I keep my focus on Jesus, the Author and Finisher of my faith. I look straight ahead, knowing Your Word is a lamp to my feet and a light to my path. If I stumble, I will not fall, for I know You will lift me up.

Reflections on the day *(write tonight or tomorrow morning in your journal).*

DAY FOURTEEN

Bible reading: Luke, chapters 10 through 13

Scripture for today (write it in your journal): "Where your treasure is, there your heart will be also" (Luke 12:34).

What does it mean? Notice Jesus didn't say "Where your heart is, there your treasure will be also." He said for us to focus on what we treasure, and we'll find what our heart truly values.

As followers of Christ, our relationship with the Lord is our dearest treasure. The presence of the Holy Spirit and the Word we've stored in our hearts are treasures we have in these "earthen vessels." Our relationships with loved ones are dear to us, but putting God first ensures all other relationships will go more smoothly. By focusing on the eternal treasure of our lives in Christ and valuing those things the Lord values, we will never be spiritually bankrupt.

Those who do not have a personal relationship with God have other treasures: people, possessions, money, power, reputation, sports, education, religion, and a host of other things to which they attach their self-worth and security.

When I was a New Ager, I shunned people who condemned me but embraced those Christians who seemed genuinely interested in me. One day a Christian man who showed appreciation for my spiritual (but non-Christian) songs said, "You know Laurette, Jesus *is* the Word of God." I was willing to listen to him because he wasn't a stranger lecturing me on my sinful lifestyle. His words reverberated in my mind for weeks, and I committed my life to the Lord shortly thereafter.

One way to show the love of God to unbelievers is to ask the Lord to reveal to you what they treasure, for then you will have a door to their heart. Show interest and side with them in the area of their treasure. Look for ways to share the good news of Jesus Christ.

Proclamation (say aloud): Jesus is my treasure and my portion forever. Thank You, Father, for sharing Your dearest treasure, Your Son, to redeem mankind and give us new life. *(Praise the Lord for who He is and for helping you speak to the hearts of others with His love.)*

What is the Lord saying to me in this Scripture? (Write it in your journal.)

Confession (start the day with a clean slate. Confess your sins, repent, and ask for God's forgiveness.)

Forgiveness (*start the day with a clean heart. In your journal, write the names of people you forgive.*)

Requests: I pray for the leaders of our nation and those in authority. I pray for the peace of Jerusalem and for the safety and effectiveness of our military at home and overseas. I now lift up the needs of my family and friends (*write your requests for others in your journal*).

I offer up my personal prayers today. Lord, I pray for Your help and guidance in these areas (*write your personal requests in your journal*).

Jesus said, "Whatever things you ask when you pray, believe that you receive them, and you will have them." I believe I receive the answer to my prayers now. Thank You, Father!

Food plan for today (*breakfast, snack, lunch, snack, dinner. Write it in your journal*).

Tummy curfew: I commit to stop eating three hours before bedtime.

Exercise plan for today (*write it in your journal*).

Top three goals for this year (*write them in your journal*).

Three things I commit to do today (*write them in your journal*).

I commit my day to the Lord. Thank You, Lord, for giving me the key into the hearts of people who are hungry and searching for You. As I go about my day today, please give me the opportunity to shine the light of Your love into their lives so they will be drawn to You.

Reflections on the day (*write tonight or tomorrow morning in your journal*).

DAY FIFTEEN

Bible reading: Luke, chapters 14 through 18

Scripture for today (*write it in your journal*): "Were there not any found who returned to give glory to God except this foreigner?... Arise, go your way. Your faith has made you well" (Luke 17:18-19).

What does it mean? In the King James Version of the ten lepers' encounter with Jesus, the Lord told the one who returned to give thanks, "Arise, go thy way: thy faith hath made thee whole." All ten were cleansed of their leprosy "as they went" in obedience to what Jesus told them to do, but one was made *completely whole* when he came back to glorify and give thanks to God. In my mind, that means all ten were healed of leprosy, but nine may still have shown the scars of their sickness. Lepers often had missing fingers, and parts of their faces and bodies were sometimes eaten away by that horrible disease. I believe the one who fell at Jesus' feet and gave thanks was totally restored without a trace of leprosy.

Thanksgiving and glorifying God bring wholeness of spirit, soul, and body. Wholeness is the Hebrew understanding of peace *(shalom):* nothing missing, nothing broken.

Our position in Christ gives us access to His peace and wholeness in every area of our lives—nothing missing, nothing broken. So, arise! Your faith in Christ has made you whole.

Proclamation *(say aloud):* I am alive in Christ! I thank You, Father God, for giving Your Son Jesus so we can experience the *shalom* of God— nothing missing, nothing broken. I delight in giving thanks to God. In fact, Father, I want to thank You for three of the biggest blessings in my life: _____, _____, and _____. *(Praise the Lord for who He is and for the blessings most of us have taken for granted.)*

What is the Lord saying to me in this Scripture? *(Write it in your journal.)*

Confession *(start the day with a clean slate. Confess your sins, repent, and ask for God's forgiveness.)*

Forgiveness *(start the day with a clean heart. In your journal, write the names of people you forgive.)*

Requests: I pray for the leaders of our nation and those in authority. I pray for the peace of Jerusalem and for the safety and effectiveness of our military at home and overseas. I now lift up the needs of my family and friends *(write your requests for others in your journal).*

I offer up my personal prayers today. Lord, I pray for Your help and guidance in these areas *(write your personal requests in your journal).*

Jesus said, "Whatever things you ask when you pray, believe that you receive them, and you will have them." I believe I receive the answer to my prayers now. Thank You, Father!

Food plan for today *(breakfast, snack, lunch, snack, dinner. Write it in your journal).*

Tummy curfew: I commit to stop eating three hours before bedtime.

Exercise plan for today *(write it in your journal).*

Top three goals for this year *(write them in your journal).*

Three things I commit to do today (write them in your journal).
I commit my day to the Lord. I will rejoice in the Lord always. I stir up thankfulness in my heart today. Lord, as I go about my day, please remind me of the many blessings in my life. I commit my will and my life to You.

Reflections on the day (write tonight or tomorrow morning in your journal).

DAY SIXTEEN

Bible reading: Luke, chapters 19 through 22

Scripture for today (write it in your journal): "And He took bread, gave thanks and broke it, and gave it to them, saying, 'This is My body which is given for you; do this in remembrance of Me.' Likewise He also took the cup after supper, saying 'This cup is the new covenant in My blood, which is shed for you'" (Luke 22:19-20).

What does it mean? Different churches celebrate communion in different ways. Some have communion every week, some once a month, others only once or twice a year. In the early church the celebration of the Lord's Supper was not an occasional event. Believers were "continuing *daily* with one accord in the temple, and breaking bread from house to house" (Acts 2:46). Communion took place in the homes on a regular basis wherever believers were present.

Paul seems to suggest there is no set schedule when we must take communion. "For *as often* as you eat this bread and drink this cup, you proclaim the Lord's death till He comes" (1 Corinthians 11:26). Proclaiming His death is also proclaiming the reason for His death and the truth of His glorious resurrection until He comes again.

If you would like to learn more about the blessing of communion, I highly recommend several resources offered by Perry Stone of Voice of Evangelism Ministries. One is his book entitled *The Meal That Heals,* which you may order at www.VoiceofEvangelism.org or by calling (423) 478-3456. A DVD and portable communion kit are also available. I take the kit with me when I travel. It is also convenient for sharing communion with a loved one in the hospital.

Proclamation (say aloud): Jesus gave His body and precious blood to redeem mankind, to deliver us from the power of darkness and sin, and to translate us into His kingdom of light and love. I am grateful beyond words for His sacrifice, and I am not ashamed of the gospel of

Christ, for it is the power of God to salvation for everyone who believes. *(Praise the Lord for who He is and for the life-giving covenant He gave us, sealed by the blood of Jesus.)*

What is the Lord saying to me in this Scripture? *(Write it in your journal.)*

Confession *(start the day with a clean slate. Confess your sins, repent, and ask for God's forgiveness.)*

Forgiveness *(start the day with a clean heart. In your journal, write the names of people you forgive.)*

Requests: I pray for the leaders of our nation and those in authority. I pray for the peace of Jerusalem and for the safety and effectiveness of our military at home and overseas. I now lift up the needs of my family and friends *(write your requests for others in your journal).*

I offer up my personal prayers today. Lord, I pray for Your help and guidance in these areas *(write your personal requests in your journal).*

Jesus said, "Whatever things you ask when you pray, believe that you receive them, and you will have them." I believe I receive the answer to my prayers now. Thank You, Father!

Food plan for today *(breakfast, snack, lunch, snack, dinner. Write it in your journal).*

Tummy curfew: I commit to stop eating three hours before bedtime.

Exercise plan for today *(write it in your journal).*

Top three goals for this year *(write them in your journal).*

Three things I commit to do today *(write them in your journal).*

I commit my day to the Lord. Lord, as I give You my day, I give thanks anew for the life You have given me in Christ. Without You I am nothing—but with You all things are possible!

Reflections on the day *(write tonight or tomorrow morning in your journal).*

DAY SEVENTEEN

Bible reading: Luke 23 through John 2

Scripture for today *(write it in your journal):* "His mother [Mary] said to the servants, 'Whatever He says to you, do it'" (John 2:5).

What does it mean? At the beginning of Jesus' ministry, Mary knew better than anyone else that her Son was more than just a man.

When the wedding hosts ran out of wine, Mary believed that her Son could help. She told Him, "They have no wine." A casual reading of Jesus' reply might cause us to think He was being insensitive or abrupt with His mother by saying, "Woman, what does your concern have to do with Me? My hour has not yet come." However, the Weymouth translation gives greater clarity and seems in keeping with the character of our Lord. " 'Leave the matter in my hands,' He replied; 'the time for me to act has not yet come.' "[24]

Immediately Mary told the servants, "Whatever He says to you, do it."

Have you found yourself asking, "When, Lord, when?" or "Why, Lord, why?" He may not seem to be acting on some pressing issue. You may wonder if He even cares. I have good news for you today. The One who measures the oceans in the hollow of His hand knows the weight of every matter that concerns you. He knows the exact moment to take action. God's timing is not our timing because His timing is always perfect.

Cast the whole of your care on the Lord today and hear Him say to you, "Leave the matter in My hands. The time for Me to act has not yet come." Then whatever He tells you to do in His Word and in your heart, do it.

Proclamation *(say aloud):* "Those who wait on the LORD shall renew their strength; they shall mount up with wings like eagles, they shall run and not be weary, they shall walk and not faint."[25] I wait on the timing of the Lord, letting patience have its perfect work in me that I may be perfect and complete, lacking nothing.[26] *(Praise the Lord for who He is, for His perfect timing, and for perfecting everything that concerns you.)*

What is the Lord saying to me in this Scripture? *(Write it in your journal.)*

Confession *(start the day with a clean slate. Confess your sins, repent, and ask for God's forgiveness.)*

Forgiveness *(start the day with a clean heart. In your journal, write the names of people you forgive.)*

Requests: I pray for the leaders of our nation and those in authority. I pray for the peace of Jerusalem and for the safety and effectiveness of our military at home and overseas. I now lift up the needs of my family and friends *(write your requests for others in your journal).*

I offer up my personal prayers today. Lord, I pray for Your help and guidance in these areas *(write your personal requests in your journal).*

Jesus said, "Whatever things you ask when you pray, believe that you receive them, and you will have them." I believe I receive the answer to my prayers now. Thank You, Father!

Food plan for today (breakfast, snack, lunch, snack, dinner. Write it in your journal).

Tummy curfew: I commit to stop eating three hours before bedtime.

Exercise plan for today (write it in your journal).

Top three goals for this year (write them in your journal).

Three things I commit to do today (write them in your journal).

I commit my day to the Lord. Lord, whatever You tell me to do, I will do. I will not race out ahead of Your perfect timing, nor will I lag behind. My life is in the safest of all possible places: Your hands.

Reflections on the day (write tonight or tomorrow morning in your journal).

DAY EIGHTEEN

Bible reading: John, chapters 3 through 6

Scripture for today (write it in your journal): "Then Jesus said to the twelve, 'Do you also want to go away?' But Simon Peter answered Him, 'Lord, to whom shall we go? You have the words of eternal life'" (John 6:67-68).

What does it mean? Jesus, the Bread of Life, had just finished teaching at the synagogue in Capernaum where He said, "Whoever eats My flesh and drinks My blood has eternal life." At this point, many men and women and their families were following Jesus. Yet when they heard this difficult teaching, many of them grumbled and were offended. From that point on, those who had only followed Jesus because of the signs and wonders He performed went back to their old lives.

New converts and immature Christians can become quickly offended. Jesus spoke of this in His parable of the sower. The seed of the word that fell on the stony ground (representing new or immature believers) sprang up quickly but withered away. There were no "roots" to their faith. They "believe for a while," Jesus said, "and in time of temptation fall away."[27]

Disciples, however, consider Jesus to be more than "fire insurance." To them He is not only Savior but also Lord and Master over *all* aspects of their lives. Peter saw more than signs and wonders when he saw Jesus. He saw the One who has "the words of eternal life." No matter how hard the sayings of Jesus were, he and the other disciples knew that no one else was like Him.

Even though they made mistakes and stumbled, the ones who continued on with Jesus bore fruit like the seed sown on good ground. "Having heard the word with a noble and good heart [they] keep it and bear fruit with patience."[28]

Proclamation (say aloud): I am a disciple of the Lord Jesus Christ. I follow Him because He has the words of eternal life. I give attention to God's words; I incline my ear to His sayings. I do not let them depart from my eyes. I keep them in the midst of my heart; for they are life to me and health to all my flesh.[29] *(Praise the Lord for who He is and for His eternal Word.)*

What is the Lord saying to me in this Scripture? (Write it in your journal.)

Confession (start the day with a clean slate. Confess your sins, repent, and ask for God's forgiveness.)

Forgiveness (start the day with a clean heart. In your journal, write the names of people you forgive.)

Requests: I pray for the leaders of our nation and those in authority. I pray for the peace of Jerusalem and for the safety and effectiveness of our military at home and overseas. I now lift up the needs of my family and friends *(write your requests for others in your journal).*

I offer up my personal prayers today. Lord, I pray for Your help and guidance in these areas *(write your personal requests in your journal).*

Jesus said, "Whatever things you ask when you pray, believe that you receive them, and you will have them." I believe I receive the answer to my prayers now. Thank You, Father!

Food plan for today (breakfast, snack, lunch, snack, dinner. Write it in your journal).

Tummy curfew: I commit to stop eating three hours before bedtime.

Exercise plan for today (write it in your journal).

Top three goals for this year (write them in your journal).

Three things I commit to do today (write them in your journal).

I commit my day to the Lord. I love You, Lord, and cherish Your words of life. I will let nothing come between us. Thank You for Your perfecting hand at work in my life today.

Reflections on the day (write tonight or tomorrow morning in your journal).

DAY NINETEEN

Bible reading: John, chapters 7 through 11

Scripture for today (write it in your journal): "If you abide in My word, you are My disciples indeed. And you shall know the truth, and the truth shall make you free" (John 8:31-32).

What does it mean? Some years ago I overheard the ultrahip young star of a popular network sitcom tell his young friend, "Hey, the truth will make ya free, man." Yeah, like wow.

That may sound deep and spiritual, but it's not only misquoting Scripture, it's incorrect. If people do not *know* the truth, the truth cannot make them free. Jesus said, "And you shall *know* the truth...." It's the truth that we come to know by abiding in the Word that makes us free.

Jesus said when praying to the Father, "Your word is truth."[30] We will know the truth by abiding (living, spending time) in the Word on a daily basis. I would be fooling myself if I said I'm abiding in a house I rarely visit. It would be equally foolish to say I'm abiding in the Word because I listen to a passage of Scripture once a week at church.

When I was a new Christian, I had so many areas of lack and bondage, I hardly knew where to begin! One area of weakness was in the area of diligence. I could start a project all right, but I had a difficult time finishing what I started. I began to study every Scripture I could find on diligence. I memorized several of them and spoke them over myself. For example, I learned that Proverbs 12:27 said that "diligence is man's precious possession." When I would be tempted to quit something that became difficult or uncomfortable, I'd tell myself, "Diligence is my precious possession." For good measure I'd say, "The hand of the diligent makes [one] rich, Laurette."[31] I quickly discovered that part of my financial problem was tied to a lack of diligence. In time I became more dependable, and our financial situation improved too.

The Word is not some magic formula, and we should not trust in vain repetition. We study, believe, speak, and act on the Word until we *know that we know* it's the truth. That's how the truth makes us free.

Proclamation (say aloud): I study to show myself approved to God, a worker who does not need to be ashamed, rightly dividing the word of truth, which sets me free.[32] *(Praise the Lord for who He is and for giving you knowledge and understanding of the truth.)*

What is the Lord saying to me in this Scripture? (Write it in your journal.)

Confession *(start the day with a clean slate. Confess your sins, repent, and ask for God's forgiveness.)*

Forgiveness *(start the day with a clean heart. In your journal, write the names of people you forgive.)*

Requests: I pray for the leaders of our nation and those in authority. I pray for the peace of Jerusalem and for the safety and effectiveness of our military at home and overseas. I now lift up the needs of my family and friends *(write your requests for others in your journal).*

I offer up my personal prayers today. Lord, I pray for Your help and guidance in these areas *(write your personal requests in your journal).*

Jesus said, "Whatever things you ask when you pray, believe that you receive them, and you will have them." I believe I receive the answer to my prayers now. Thank You, Father!

Food plan for today *(breakfast, snack, lunch, snack, dinner. Write it in your journal).*

Tummy curfew: I commit to stop eating three hours before bedtime.

Exercise plan for today *(write it in your journal).*

Top three goals for this year *(write them in your journal).*

Three things I commit to do today *(write them in your journal).*

I commit my day to the Lord. I pray to know Your truth more fully every day.

Reflections on the day *(write tonight or tomorrow morning in your journal).*

DAY TWENTY

Bible reading: John, chapters 12 through 16

Scripture for today *(write it in your journal):* "I am the vine, you are the branches. He who abides in Me, and I in him, bears much fruit; for without Me you can do nothing" (John 15:5).

What does it mean? Just as branches cannot bear fruit without their vine, a vine cannot bear fruit without the branches.

What is the fruit of the Christian life? We have discussed the fruit of the Spirit being developed in our lives (love, joy, peace, patience, kindness, goodness, faithfulness, gentleness, and self-control[33]). We also bear fruit by leading others to the Lord[34] and by giving aid and finances to help others.[35] The sacrifice of praise to God is offering "the fruit of our lips."[36] Good works and meeting the needs of others for the glory of God also bear fruit.[37]

The beauty of bearing fruit in the Lord's vineyard is that the harvest is continual, not seasonal. The fruit is not short-lived, nor does it wither and die. The fruit we bear by abiding in the vine is eternal. Jesus said, "And he who reaps receives wages, and gathers fruit for eternal life, that both he who sows and he who reaps may rejoice together" (John 4:36).

Perhaps you have been sowing seeds of love and service into the lives of others for years without seeing the fruit of your labors. You may wonder if that young man or young woman you witnessed to all those years ago ever came to the Lord. The good news is that eternal fruit never dies—the one who sows and the one who reaps will rejoice together—so rejoice!

Proclamation *(say aloud):* I am a branch of the living vine, Jesus Christ. I abide in Him, and He abides in me. Together we bear much fruit. Without Him I can do nothing, but with Him all things are possible! *(Praise the Lord for who He is and for the opportunities He gives you to sow seeds into the lives of others, yielding eternal fruit for God's kingdom.)*

What is the Lord saying to me in this Scripture? *(Write it in your journal.)*

Confession *(start the day with a clean slate. Confess your sins, repent, and ask for God's forgiveness.)*

Forgiveness *(start the day with a clean heart. In your journal, write the names of people you forgive.)*

Requests: I pray for the leaders of our nation and those in authority. I pray for the peace of Jerusalem and for the safety and effectiveness of our military at home and overseas. I now lift up the needs of my family and friends *(write your requests for others in your journal).*

I offer up my personal prayers today. Lord, I pray for Your help and guidance in these areas *(write your personal requests in your journal).*

Jesus said, "Whatever things you ask when you pray, believe that you receive them, and you will have them." I believe I receive the answer to my prayers now. Thank You, Father!

Food plan for today *(breakfast, snack, lunch, snack, dinner. Write it in your journal).*

Tummy curfew: I commit to stop eating three hours before bedtime.

Exercise plan for today (write it in your journal).

Top three goals for this year (write them in your journal).

Three things I commit to do today (write them in your journal).

I commit my day to the Lord. Lord, help me realize that this is not just another day. Every day in You is an adventure. I am vitally connected to You, and as Your branch I reach out to touch the lives of others with Your message of love and hope. I love You, Jesus. Let's go out and gather some fruit for eternal life today!

Reflections on the day (write tonight or tomorrow morning in your journal).

DAY TWENTY-ONE

Bible reading: John, chapters 17 through 21

Scripture for today (write it in your journal): "Thomas, because you have seen Me, you have believed. Blessed are those who have not seen and yet have believed" (John 20:29).

What does it mean? God's Word tells us, "The just shall live by faith,"[38] yet many of us still live by what we see and feel. Feelings are fleeting. What is seen is only temporary.

The Weymouth translation of Hebrews 11:3 states, "Through faith we understand that the worlds came into being, and still exist, at the command of God, so that what is seen does not owe its existence to that which is visible." What we see is made of the substance of faith, so it is vital to our existence to become conversant in the language of faith contained in the Word of God.

Those who believe in what they have not yet seen are blessed because their faith is based on something higher than physical circumstances. Facts are subject to change. Truth is higher than facts and cannot be changed. What science may call "magical thinking," Christianity calls faith. It is the *substance* of things hoped for and the *evidence* of things not seen.

My favorite definition of *blessed* is this: empowered to break through to success. Jesus is saying that when you believe, you are blessed. You are *empowered by God* to break through to success in every area of your life. The Amplified Bible in 1 Chronicles 14:11 calls God "the Lord of breaking through." Breakthrough is His specialty. He will not let you be ashamed that you put your trust in Him. "For the eyes of the Lord run to and fro throughout the whole earth, to show Himself strong on behalf of those whose heart is loyal to Him."[39] You cannot fail!

Proclamation *(say aloud):* Jesus said I am blessed because I believe even though I have not fully seen. Being blessed, I am empowered by God to break through to success. I'm stepping up and stepping out in faith. I am stronger than I was 21 days ago. With God all things are possible. Hallelujah! *(Praise God for who He is and for being the Lord of your breakthrough!)*

What is the Lord saying to me in this Scripture? *(Write it in your journal.)*

Confession *(start the day with a clean slate. Confess your sins, repent, and ask for God's forgiveness.)*

Forgiveness *(start the day with a clean heart. In your journal, write the names of people you forgive.)*

Requests: I pray for the leaders of our nation and those in authority. I pray for the peace of Jerusalem and for the safety and effectiveness of our military at home and overseas. I now lift up the needs of my family and friends *(write your requests for others in your journal).*

I offer up my personal prayers today. Lord, I pray for Your help and guidance in these areas *(write your personal requests in your journal).*

Jesus said, "Whatever things you ask when you pray, believe that you receive them, and you will have them." I believe I receive the answer to my prayers now. Thank You, Father!

Food plan for today *(breakfast, snack, lunch, snack, dinner. Write it in your journal).*

Tummy curfew: I commit to stop eating three hours before bedtime.

Exercise plan for today *(write it in your journal).*

Top three goals for this year *(write them in your journal).*

Three things I commit to do today *(write them in your journal).*

I commit my day to the Lord. Lord, I trust You to help me continue to develop these healthier new habits I've been walking in the last few weeks. My body is the temple of Your Holy Spirit, and it is my joy to glorify You in my body and in my spirit, which are Yours.

Reflections on the day *(write tonight or tomorrow morning in your journal).*

11

BASIC Steps Recipes

KISS (Keep It Simple, Sweetheart) Meals

Breakfast: Eggs are a good source of protein and can be prepared a number of ways. Look for "cage-free" eggs or those with the USDA Organic label, which means that neither the hens nor their feed have been subjected to antibiotics, hormones, pesticides, or herbicides.

- Vegetable omelets are a quick and easy meal any time of day—just add your favorite veggies.

- Eggs can be scrambled, hard- or soft-boiled, or poached.

- Quiche—how about a Quick Quiche (see the recipes later in this chapter) for dinner and leftovers for breakfast or lunch the next day?

- Cereal—use whole grain cereals, brown rice, oatmeal, or rye with almond milk or skim milk.

- Choose whole wheat or Ezekiel 4:9 bagels, bread, or English muffins with all-fruit jam.

- If you are eating a carbohydrate-rich breakfast or lunch (grains and breads, for example), slow the release of sugar into the bloodstream by adding a small amount of nuts or seeds (such as almonds, walnuts, macadamia

nuts, or sunflower seeds). The good fat content found
in nuts and seeds can help prevent blood sugar imbalances by slowing the uptake of sugar into the bloodstream.

- Coming off coffee? Ask at your health food store for
  Teeccino, a caffeine-free herbal coffee (I like Hazel-
  nut—yum!). Postum is available at your grocer's.

Lunch: Protein-rich meals with a big veggie salad will ensure stamina throughout the afternoon without that mid-afternoon slump
from overdoing carbs at lunchtime. Combining different sources of
protein in a salad (without loading up on fatty, chemical-laden salad
dressings) is a smart choice for a high-powered lunch. Choose eggs,
chicken, turkey, fish, or soy.

- Warmed whole wheat tortillas stuffed with avocado,
  broccoli-slaw, shredded cheese (dairy, soy, or rice cheese),
  tomatoes, spinach leaves, and salsa is one of our favorite
  home lunches.

- Put one or two hard-boiled eggs in a big leafy green
  salad with veggies.

- Make homemade vegetable soup with bits of chicken
  or soy burger.

- Sandwiches are great with chicken, egg, or tuna salad
  (light on the mayo), spinach leaves, romaine, or green
  leaf lettuce, and on whole grain bread, or Ezekiel 4:9
  bread, or rolls.

- Eating out? Eat as many whole, unprocessed foods as
  possible for maximum fitness and energy. The salad bar
  is a great choice. Just remember your portion sizes
  (small handful), load up on the greens, and go light on
  the dressing.

- Enjoy tortillas, enchiladas, fajitas, or quesadillas (with
  meat, but go light on the cheese) with beans. Avoid
  white rice and fried tortilla chips.

- Practice "God's Heavenly Weigh" (leave some food on
  your plate).

Brown Bag Tips: Prepare lunches the night before to avoid the last-minute morning rush. For children, limit portion sizes to avoid waste (½ cup servings, ½ sandwich, a few fruit slices instead of the whole fruit, and baby carrots). Provide a vegetable and a protein with each meal (proteins include lean meats, soy products, grains, beans, nut butters, and seeds). Put a sugar-free treat in each lunch (fruit, applesauce, raisins, a homemade cookie, or a muffin). Keep moist sandwich ingredients in a separate container to avoid soggy sandwiches.

Dinner: The old saying is really sound fitness advice: Eat the breakfast of a king, the lunch of a prince, and the dinner of a pauper. Let dinner be your smallest meal of the day. Eat more protein and less carbs at dinner if you want to lose weight.

- Remember the "Tummy Curfew." Do not eat within three hours of bedtime.

- Many of the lunch suggestions will also work for dinner. Even some breakfast items make a nourishing dinner, such as an omelet or quiche with a side salad of veggies and brown rice.

- Stir-fry veggies with a little olive oil and a protein source (soy crumbles, chicken, or fish); serve with whole wheat pasta or brown rice and salad. Don't forget to add those fresh sprouts!

- Serve chili (with or without meat) with brown or basmati rice and lightly steamed or raw veggies.

- Enjoy chicken and whole wheat pasta with salad.

- Try turkey burgers with baked sweet potato and shredded cabbage-carrot slaw.

- Seasoning—avoid table salt and use sea salt or seasonings without MSG (such as Mrs. Dash). Experiment with fresh herbs from the supermarket—or grow your own!

Desserts and Snacks: Retrain your taste buds to enjoy the natural sweetness of fresh fruit without sugar and artificial sweeteners.

- Garnish fresh fruit salad with a sprig of mint.

- NatraLean bars from NatraTech are wonderful. These low-glycemic, hypoallergenic nutrition bars have no dairy products, corn, peanuts, soy, wheat, or sugar. Dr. Lopez also has great supplements for adrenal support, a free stress test, a free nutritional eating plan to download, and additional info at www.NatraTech.com. Mention Laurette Willis and save 10 percent or more.

- Instead of chocolate, ask for carob powder or carob chips at your health food store (it's sometimes called St. John's Bread). Carob is similar to chocolate but without the sugar or caffeine. We also enjoy Wondercocoa powder by Wonderslim. It's made from 100 percent roasted cocoa beans, and it's sugar free and caffeine free (tastes great in smoothies!)

- Peel a banana, cut it into slices, and freeze it. I enjoy this treat with grain-sweetened carob chips. A variation of this is to dip a banana in melted carob chips, place it on wax paper, and freeze it. Poke a popsicle stick into one end of the banana for a delectable banana-carob pop.

- Wash and freeze grapes for an icy treat on a hot day.

- Smoothies make a filling and healthful snack (see the recipes below).

- Remember to make healthful foods convenient. Keep a big bowl of apples, oranges, bananas, and fruits in season on the kitchen counter. Remove all substandard "dead" foods from your cupboards and refrigerator. You're not throwing money away—you're investing in your health.

Time-Savers

- Plan your meals for the week and buy the ingredients ahead of time.

- Spend an hour on the weekend cooking—freeze individual portions and reheat them later.

- Double or triple a recipe and freeze the rest.

- Cook something on the weekend that will give you leftovers for a casserole.

- Frozen veggies are the next best thing to fresh. Bags of assorted veggies make a quick stir-fry.

- Don't go shopping without a list. Create a computer file of everything you normally purchase and put a line next to each item. You only have to do this once. Print it out each week and put it on the refrigerator. As you run out of an item, any member of the family can put a checkmark next to it on the list. Your list can include not only food items but soap and paper products as well. It could keep you from making several trips to the store during the week.

Help! My Kids *Hate* Veggies!

No problem! Disguise them (the veggies that is, not the kids!). Finely dice carrots, tomatoes, and bell peppers into spaghetti sauce. Make muffins with shredded pieces of zucchini and carrots. Sauté diced vegetables to soften them, and add them to meatballs or turkey burgers. Add chopped broccoli, cauliflower, and carrots to pizza and cover with grated cheese and sauce. Puree veggies and add to soup or stew—it will look just like part of the broth. Mix grated or pureed vegetables into their pancakes, peanut or almond butter—even macaroni and cheese or lasagna. Increase the fiber content of your meals by adding brown rice or barley to your sauces, soups, salads, and casseroles. Disguise nutrition in a pizza by spreading pureed veggies on a pita round with sauce, sprinkle it with cheese, and broil it. Voilá!

Breakfast Recipes

BASIC Power Shake

    12 ounces water
    1 or 2 scoops protein powder (from whey, rice, soy, or egg whites)
    8 frozen strawberries (or fruit of choice)
    1 tablespoon raw almond butter (or 1 tablespoon flaxseed oil)
    1 or 2 scoops concentrated greens powder (see "Resources")
    ½ teaspoon glyconutrient powder (see "Resources")
    1 teaspoon psyllium seed husks

Combine ingredients in a blender and mix for 30 seconds. (Note: If you have digestive problems or food sensitivities, don't use dairy-based whey protein or add fruit to your protein shake. Select from the other forms of protein, and use several ice cubes instead of the frozen fruit. You can make a fruit smoothie shake without the protein or almond butter if you'd prefer.)

Tropical Breakfast or Snack

> ½ cup low-fat yogurt or cottage cheese
>
> pineapple chunks or sliced peaches without sugar
>
> 1 tablespoon real maple syrup

Orangey French Toast

> 4 egg whites
>
> ½ cup almond milk (or soy, rice, or skim milk)
>
> 2 tablespoons frozen orange juice concentrate
>
> 1 teaspoon vanilla extract
>
> ½ teaspoon cinnamon
>
> 4 slices whole grain bread
>
> ½ to 1 tablespoon all-fruit jam or real maple syrup

Gently beat egg whites. Mix egg whites, milk, frozen orange juice, vanilla, and cinnamon. Dip bread slices in liquid one at a time. Coat a skillet with nonstick cooking spray and preheat. Place each slice in skillet and cook on each side to brown. Serve topped with jam or maple syrup.

Banana Cakes

> 1 ripe banana
>
> 1 egg
>
> ½ cup whole wheat flour
>
> 2 teaspoons baking powder
>
> ½ teaspoon natural maple or vanilla flavoring

A different way to make pancakes! Blend the banana, egg, and flavoring, and then add flour and baking powder. Spoon mixture onto hot skillet coated with nonstick spray. When bubbly, turn pancakes over.

Spicy Scrambles

> 3 eggs beaten (with a few tablespoons of water)
>
> salsa sauce
>
> grated cheese (dairy, soy, rice, or almond cheese)
>
> veggies of choice

Coat skillet with nonstick cooking spray. Add eggs, scrambling them as they cook. Spread salsa on top, add cheese and veggies. Option: Cover and let cook another minute or two. Fold in half like an omelet.

Lunch Recipes

Pizza Pockets

> 1 whole wheat pita pocket (cut in half around the circle, making two pita circles)
>
> 2 tablespoons no-sugar spaghetti sauce
>
> assorted veggies (freshly cut broccoli, mushrooms, cauliflower)
>
> 1/3 to 1/2 cup shredded mozzarella cheese (nonfat dairy, soy, or rice milk cheese)

Preheat oven to 375 degrees. Place pita rounds on baking sheet and spread each with half the sauce and cheese. Bake for about 10 minutes. Serve with salad.

Chili on the Go

> 1 can of beans (black, kidney, or pinto beans)
>
> chopped tomato
>
> 1/2 teaspoon chili powder
>
> salsa to taste

Heat ingredients together. Top with grated cheese (dairy, soy, or rice milk cheese). Keep warm in a Thermos and serve with crackers and apple slices.

Egg Salad

> 4 cut-up hard-boiled eggs
>
> 2 stalks chopped celery
>
> 1/4 cup diced red onion
>
> 1/4 cup minced parsley
>
> 3 to 4 tablespoons low-fat mayonnaise (or soy mayonnaise)
>
> 1 teaspoon turmeric
>
> 1/2 to 1 teaspoon sea salt
>
> 2 tablespoons apple cider vinegar

Mix all ingredients and serve on top of salad, in a whole wheat pita pocket, wrapped into a tortilla with lettuce or spinach leaves, or as a sandwich on whole grain bread.

Finger-Lickin' Chicken Salad

> 1 cup cooked chicken pieces (use hormone-free chicken)
>
> 1 stalk chopped celery
>
> 2 diced scallions (green onions)
>
> 1/4 cup minced parsley
>
> 2 or 3 tablespoons low-fat mayonnaise (or soy mayonnaise)
>
> 1 teaspoon spicy deli mustard
>
> 1 teaspoon tamari sauce (or Bragg Liquid Aminos)
>
> 2 tablespoons pickle relish (optional)

Combine chicken, veggies, and relish in a mixing bowl. In a separate bowl, combine the mayonnaise, mustard, and tamari sauce. Combine the contents of both bowls. Chill for one hour and serve on salad or in a sandwich.

Dinner Recipes

Quiche and Tell

> 1 whole wheat pie crust
>
> 3 large eggs
>
> 1 tablespoon butter or olive oil

½ cup minced onion

1 cup nonfat milk (or soy, rice, or almond milk)

2 tablespoons nonfat dry milk powder   ·

½ teaspoon sea salt

freshly ground pepper to taste

¼ cup grated Gruyère or Jarlsberg cheese

¼ cup grated Parmesan cheese

Optional: chopped broccoli, cauliflower, mushrooms, spinach, and/or carrots

Preheat the oven to 375 degrees. Brush the pie crust with some beaten egg and bake for 7 minutes. Take out of oven and cool. Heat the butter or oil in a skillet and add onion, stirring for about 5 minutes until tender. Remove from heat. In a bowl blend the milk and powdered milk. Add sea salt, eggs, and pepper. Stir in onions and cheese. Pour into the pie crust. Bake for 30 to 40 minutes, checking to see the quiche mixture is set and the top is turning to a golden brown. Remove and let sit to cool. Serve hot or warm. Warm leftover quiche for breakfast, or take it with you for a tasty lunch with a side salad.

Sloppy Josephine

1 pound lean ground beef (or ground turkey or tofu crumbles)

½ cup chopped onion

¼ cup chopped green pepper

¼ teaspoon garlic powder

1 teaspoon mustard

¾ cup sugar-free ketchup

3 teaspoons brown sugar (or 2 packets stevia powder)

sea salt and ground black pepper to taste

whole wheat hamburger buns

Brown the ground meat, onion, and green pepper in a skillet over medium heat. Drain liquids. Mix in garlic, mustard, ketchup, and brown sugar (or stevia) and stir well. Lower heat and simmer for 30 minutes. Season with sea salt and ground pepper. Serve over whole wheat buns.

Rita's Tortilla Pizza

> 4 whole wheat tortillas
>
> 1 jar pizza sauce
>
> 8 ounces shredded low-fat mozzarella cheese
>
> favorite pizza toppings: mushrooms, black olives, onion, tomatoes…

Preheat oven to 350 degrees. Spread 3 tablespoons pizza sauce on each tortilla; top with cheese. Spray cookie sheet with nonstick cooking spray. Place pizzas on cookie sheet and bake for 5 to 8 minutes until cheese is bubbly and brown.

Sunflowered Green Beans

> 1 ½ pounds green beans, trimmed
>
> 2 tablespoons olive oil
>
> ¼ cup dry-roasted sunflower seeds (or other nuts or seeds)
>
> 2 minced garlic cloves
>
> 10 chopped basil leaves
>
> sea salt and ground pepper to taste

Steam green beans until tender but still crisp (about 7 minutes). Place green beans in a bowl of ice water to cool. Drain and dry with paper towels. Heat oil in a skillet over medium heat. Add dry-roasted sunflower seeds and brown (about 5 minutes). Add garlic and green beans. Sauté for 5 minutes. Mix in basil leaves, salt, and pepper.

Pollo (Chicken) Parmesan

> ½ cup whole wheat bread crumbs
>
> ¼ cup grated Parmesan cheese
>
> ½ teaspoon garlic powder
>
> ¼ teaspoon sea salt
>
> 1 or 2 tablespoons olive oil
>
> 1 ¼ pounds thinly sliced chicken breasts (boneless, skinless)
>
> 1 cup no-sugar spaghetti sauce (optional: add 2 teaspoons salsa to sauce)
>
> 1 cup shredded part-skim mozzarella cheese

Preheat oven to 425 degrees. Combine bread crumbs, Parmesan cheese, garlic powder, and sea salt in a bowl. Brush each chicken cutlet with olive oil and then dip in the bread crumb mixture. Spray baking sheet with nonstick cooking spray and arrange chicken on the sheet. Bake 12 to 15 minutes. Pour spaghetti sauce over the chicken, add mozzarella cheese, and bake an additional 5 to 7 minutes until the cheese has melted.

SpaghettiOs!

> 1 spaghetti squash
>
> 2 cups no-sugar spaghetti sauce
>
> 1 cup sliced mushrooms
>
> 2 tablespoons chopped parsley
>
> 2 tablespoons Parmesan cheese

Preheat oven to 400 degrees. Wash the outside of the squash and cut in half lengthwise. Remove seeds. Place squash cut side down in a shallow baking dish. Add 1 or 2 inches of water. Bake for 45 to 55 minutes until tender. Cool slightly. Heat spaghetti sauce and mushrooms. Scrape the insides of the squash with a fork to make spaghetti-like strands. Place the "spaghetti" in a bowl, add the spaghetti sauce mixture, and sprinkle with parsley and Parmesan cheese. Serve with Italian bread and salad or as a side with *Pollo Parmesan.*

Black Bean Burgers

> 1 15-ounce can of black beans, drained and mashed
>
> ¼ cup shredded carrots
>
> ½ cup corn
>
> ½ cup diced onion
>
> ½ teaspoon sea salt
>
> 4 eggs
>
> ¼ cup whole wheat bread crumbs
>
> olive oil to coat pan

Mix all ingredients; heat oil in the pan. Shape the mixture into patties and cook thoroughly on each side. Serve with mashed avocado and salsa on whole wheat buns.

Smoothies and Ice Dreams

Almond-Cocoa Smoothie

     1 cup crushed ice

     1 banana

     1 tablespoon carob powder

     2 tablespoons almond butter

     1 cup almond milk (or skim, rice, or soy milk)

     2 scoops concentrated greens powder (see "Resources")

     1 cup distilled water

Combine in blender until smooth.

Yogurt-Berry Smoothie

     1 cup crushed ice

     1 cup vanilla yogurt

     ½ cup each fresh or frozen strawberries and blueberries

     ½ banana

     1 ½ to 2 cups distilled water

Combine in blender until smooth.

Ice Dreams

Peel 2 bananas and cut into thin slices. Freeze slices overnight in a freezer bag. Put half the slices in a blender with ¼ cup of almond milk (or rice or soy milk). Blend, adding the rest of the banana slices a little at a time. Add strawberries, blueberries, peaches, or whatever fruit you prefer. Serve in chilled parfait dishes with a sprig of mint—or low-sugar waffle cones!

You can find additional recipes at www.BasicSteps.info.

A Prayer to Receive
Jesus Christ
as Your Savior

Dear God in Heaven,

I come to You in the name of Jesus. Your Word says "the one who comes to Me I will by no means cast out."[1] So I know You want to take me in, and I thank You for that.

Your Word says, "If you confess with your mouth the Lord Jesus and believe in your heart that God has raised Him from the dead, you will be saved.... For whoever calls on the name of the LORD shall be saved."[2]

I believe in my heart that Jesus is the Son of God. I believe He was raised from the dead. I confess out loud that Jesus is Lord. I am calling on the name of the Lord—I am calling on Jesus—so I know I am now saved. Thank You for helping me to receive everlasting life from You right this moment!

I believe in my heart and I confess with my mouth that Jesus is the Lord of my life. I am saved! I am a new creation in Christ Jesus. I'm a Christian, and Jesus is in my heart.

Thank You, Father!

Signed _____

Date _____

Action Steps for the New Christian:

1. Go to a Bible-believing church. A church is where you will learn how to live the Christian life and where the pastor, spiritual leaders, and Christian friends can help you and encourage you in your faith.

2. Be baptized in water in obedience to the Word of God (Matthew 28:19; Acts 2:38).

3. Read your Bible every day. Start with the Gospel of John. Get a version of the Bible you can understand and ask the Holy Spirit to reveal the Bible's truth and power to you. (The precious Holy Spirit is the Teacher and Comforter, and He now lives in your heart!)

4. Pray every day. No need to use fancy words! Simply speak to and fellowship with your Father God. He will answer your prayers and give you specific guidance to help you.

5. Strive to live a holy life. We are not perfect. We do, however, turn from the old sinful ways and seek to live in accordance with the Bible.

Resources

To keep things simple and information updated, Laurette has a website listing product and nutrition recommendations, fitness information, recipes, and updates.

Simply go to www.BasicSteps.info. There you will also find information about the *Gimme Ten Workout*™ video and DVD, *Scripture-to-Music* CDs (Scriptures set to upbeat praise music for workouts and walking, or beautiful praise hymns for stretches and relaxing), *Great Women of the Bible* CD and video (Laurette's one-woman musical drama), "A Daily Walk with the Lord's Prayer" cards, as well as nutritional product information (concentrated greens powder, glyconutrients, other dietary supplements, water purification systems, and more).

If you would like Laurette to visit your church, women's conference, school, or community organization for a Fitness for His Witness™ Seminar, PraiseMoves™ workshop, keynote address, or one of her one-woman shows (such as *Great Women of the Bible*), please visit www.LauretteWillis.com or e-mail her at Laurette@LauretteWillis.com.

Information on PraiseMoves™ products and the PraiseMoves Teacher Certification program is available at www.PraiseMoves.com.

Notes

Bad News, Good News

1. "Statistics Related to Overweight and Obesity," National Institute of Diabetes and Digestive and Kidney Diseases (NIDDK) of the National Institutes of Health (NIH). Accessed at win.niddk.nih.gov/statistics/index.htm on November 22, 2004.

2. "WELCOA Responds to the Obesity Epidemic of America," Wellness Council of America. Accessed at www.welcoa.org/freeresources/pdg/Obesity_Report.pdf on December 6, 2004.

3. 2 Peter 1:3

4. "Jesus said to him, 'I am the way, the truth and the life'" (John 14:6).

5. Matthew 19:26

Introduction

1. 2 Corinthians 12:10

2. Deuteronomy 30:19-20 NIV

3. Psalm 37:23 NIV

4. 1 Corinthians 6:20

5. 1 Thessalonians 5:23 NLT

6. Romans 8:10 NLT

7. Hebrews 4:12

8. 1 Corinthians 6:19-20 NLT

9. Acts 17:28

Chapter 1—Eating What's *Right* Will Solve What's *Wrong*

1. Galatians 6:7

2. Mark 12:30-31

3. A. Bloch, et al., "Position of the American Dietetic Association: Phytochemicals and Functional Foods," *Journal of the American Dietetic Association* 95 (1995), 493-96.

4. Melanie Polk, "Feast on Phytochemicals," *AICR Newsletter* 51 (1996).

5. Hosea 4:6

6. John 6:35

7. T.L. Davidson and S.E. Swithers, "A Pavlovian Approach to the Problem of Obesity," *International Journal of Obesity* 28 (July 2004), 933-35.

8. D.S. Ludwig, et al., "Relation Between Consumption of Sugar-Sweetened Drinks and Childhood Obesity," *The Lancet* 357 (2001), 505-08

Chapter 2—*Break*fast! It's a Command

1. J.O. Hill, et al., "The Role of Breakfast in the Treatment of Obesity," *American Journal of Clinical Nutrition* 55, no. 3 (March 1992), 645-51

2. Leviticus 23:9-11; Deuteronomy 26:1-10

3. 1 Corinthians 10:11

4. 1 Corinthians 5:7

5. Romans 12:1

6. Hebrews 13:15

7. Romans 11:16

8. Colossians 3:23

Chapter 3—Success Strategies

1. Ancel Keys, et al., "The Diet and 15 Year Death Rate in the Seven Countries Study," *American Journal of Epidemiology*, 124, no. 6 (1986), 903-15.

2. M. Flynn, "Serum Lipids and Eggs," *Journal of the American Dietetic Association* 86, no. 11 (November 1986), 1541-42

3. Don Colbert, M.D., *What Would Jesus Eat?* (Nashville: Nelson Books, 2002), 47-70.

4. David Macht, "An Experimental Pharmacological Appreciation of Leviticus XI and Deuteronomy XIV," *Bulletin of Historical Medicine*, 47, no. 1 (April 1953), 444-50

5. Leviticus 19:26

6. Jane Cahill and Peter Warnock, "It Had to Happen, Scientist Examines Ancient Bathrooms of Romans 586 B.C.," *Biblical Archeological Review* (May/June 1991).

7. Galatians 5:16

8. Colossians 3:23-24

9. 2 Corinthians 9:6

10. Philippians 4:13

11. James 4:2

12. R.H. Fletcher and K.M. Fairfeld, "Vitamins for Chronic Disease Prevention in Adults," *Journal of the American Medical Association* 278, no. 23 (2002), 3127-29.

13. H.J. Montoye, et al., *Measuring Physical Activity and Energy Expenditure,* (Champaign, IL: Human Kinetics Publishers, 1996), 97-115.

14. "Common Nutrients for a Common Condition," in *Prevention's Healing with Vitamins,* ed. Alice Feinstein (Emmaus, PA: Rodale Books, 1998). Accessed online at www.mothernature.com/Library/Bookshelf/Books/10/48.cfm on September 16, 2004.

15. B.H. McAnalley and E. Vennum, "Introduction to Glyconutritionals," *Glycoscience & Nutrition Journal* 1, no. 1 (2000) 1-5.

16. Thomas H. Gardiner, et. al., *Choices: Choosing the Right Dietary Supplements for Optimal Health* (Grand Prairie, TX: Talking Stick Publishing Corporation, 2004), 15-38.

Chapter 4—Movement: Are You Sitting Down?

1. 1 Timothy 4:8

2. Ibid.

3. Romans 12:1

4. 1 Corinthians 6:19-20

5. Philippians 4:8

6. Ephesians 6:17

7. Based on Philippians 4:13; Ephesians 6:10; Romans 8:37

8. Proverbs 4:22

9. James 1:5

10. Ephesians 4:27 NIV

11. Nehemiah 8:10

12. Matthew 6:7-9

13. Psalm 122:6

14. 1 Timothy 2:1-2

15. Philippians 4:19; 2 Peter 1:3

16. Psalm 5:12

17. Malachi 3:10; Proverbs 19:17; Luke 6:38

18. 1 John 1:9

19. Romans 13:8

20. Exodus 12:23-25

21. Ephesians 6:10-17

22. Psalm 91:11

23. John 10:4,27

24. Philippians 4:13

25. Psalm 3:3

26. Psalm 23:1

27. Mark 10:27

28. Hebrews 10:38

29. Proverbs 4:7

30. Psalm 27:1

31. 2 Timothy 1:7

32. John 10:10

33. Galatians 3:13

34. Philippians 4:19

35. Luke 6:38

Chapter 5—Renewing Your Mind: Where Godly Fitness Begins

1. Psalm 34:19

2. Ephesians 5:1

3. Romans 10:17

4. Hebrews 11:1

5. Spiros Zodhiates, *The Complete WordStudy New Testament* (Chattanooga, TN: AMG Publishers, 1992), 964.

6. 1 Corinthians 9:27 NLT

7. Luke 16:10

8. James 1:17

9. 1 John 1:9

10. Isaiah 54:17

11. 2 Corinthians 10:4 AMP

12. Ephesians 1:6

13. Philippians 4:13

14. Mark 11:24

15. Philippians 4:8

16. Colossians 3:1-2

17. Romans 12:2 NLT

18. Romans 14:23

19. Proverbs 4:20-22

20. Matthew 4:4

21. 1 Corinthians 10:13

22. James 2:26

23. 2 Corinthians 4:18

24. 2 Peter 1:3

25. Joel 2:26-27

26. Luke 17:14

27. Romans 12:2

Chapter 6—Emotions: Forgiveness, the Key to Answered Prayer

1. Mark 11:25-26

2. 1 Corinthians 11:27-31

3. Isaiah 42:3 NIV

4. Isaiah 61:3

5. Matthew 9:36

6. Galatians 5:6

7. 1 John 4:8

Chapter 7—Stress: America's Number One Health Problem

1. Psalm 31:15

2. Galatians 3:13

3. 1 Peter 5:6-7

4. Philippians 4:6

5. 1 John 5:14-15

6. John 1:3

7. Psalm 37:4

8. Hebrews 4:9-11

Chapter 8—Prayer, Praise and Fasting: God's Power Tools

1. Luke 11:1

2. Psalm 103:12

3. Isaiah 43:25

4. Hebrews 13:15

5. The word translated as "bring" in Hebrew is '*âlâh,* which means "ascend." There is no distinction in Hebrew between the causative and the permissive tenses of a verb. Since *ascend* means to bring up from below and God is above, many scholars see this as God *permitting* calamity from the enemy, not causing it.

6. Matthew 6:7

7. Proverbs 4:22

8. 1 Kings 19:12

9. Mark 11:24

10. 1 John 5:14-15

11. 2 Corinthians 4:18

12. Hebrews 11:1

13. John 10:4

14. Ephesians 6:12

15. 1 Peter 5:8

16. Isaiah 26:3

17. Acts 16:25 KJV

18. Isaiah 58:6

19. Matthew 6:16

Chapter 9—PraiseMoves: The Christian Alternative to Yoga

1. Romans 8:14; John 10:4

2. Sarah E. Pavlik, "Is Yoga Really So Bad?" *Today's Christian Woman,* 23, no. 5 (September/October 2001), 50.

3. Ibid.

4. Romans 3:23-25 NLT

5. Proverbs 8:12 KJV

6. "Exercise Tips: Weight Control," *The Fit Society* (January–March 2001), 8.

7. 1 Corinthians 6:19, 1 John 4:4

8. Hebrews 12:2

9. 1 Corinthians 6:20

10. Laura DeMarco, "The Yoga Evolution: Old Practice Leads to Big Business with New Twists," *The Plain Dealer* (August 2, 2004). Accessed online at www. cleveland.com on September 6, 2004.

Chapter 10—The Step-UP Program: 21 Days to a Not-So-Extreme Makeover by God's Design

1. 1 Timothy 2:1-2

2. Psalm 122:6-9

3. Mark 11:24

4. Habakkuk 2:4; Romans 1:17; Galatians 3:11; Hebrews 10:38

5. 2 Corinthians 5:21

6. Hebrews 11:6

7. 2 Corinthians 3:18

8. Psalm 19:14

9. Matthew 9:22; Mark 5:34; 10:52; Luke 8:48; 17:19

10. Mark 6:5-6

11. Hebrews 4:16

12. 2 Corinthians 10:5

13. 2 Corinthians 2:11

14. Ephesians 3:16

15. 1 Peter 5:6-7

16. Mark 10:27

17. 1 John 4:8,16

18. John 3:16

19. Galatians 5:6

20. 1 John 4:18

21. 1 Corinthians 13:8

22. Luke 17:32 (Jesus is referring to Genesis 19:26. Lot's wife looked back at the destruction of Sodom and Gomorrah and turned into a pillar of salt.)

23. 2 Corinthians 9:8

24. John 2:4, Weymouth New Testament in Modern English

25. Isaiah 40:31

26. James 1:4

27. Luke 8:13

28. Luke 8:15

29. Proverbs 4:20-22

30. John 17:17

31. Proverbs 10:4

32. 2 Timothy 2:15

33. Galatians 5:22

34. John 4:35-36

35. Philippians 4:17

36. Hebrews 13:15

37. Titus 3:14

38. Habakkuk 2:4; Romans 1:17; Galatians 3:11; Hebrews 10:38

39. 2 Chronicles 16:9

A Prayer to Receive Jesus Christ as Your Savior

1. John 6:37

2. Romans 10:9,13

Other Good
Harvest House Reading

LOVE TO EAT, HATE TO EAT
Elyse Fitzpatrick

Not just another diet book, Elyse Fitzpatrick helps women make realistic, practical steps toward proper eating, health, and emotional balance. With biblical guidelines for victory, this book is ideal for Christian women who want to fully yield this area of their lives to the Lord.

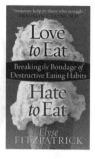

GREATER HEALTH GOD'S WAY
Stormie Omartian

For everyone who has tried diet programs, only to find them less than completely satisfying, bestselling author Stormie Omartian provides a creative, practical approach to developing a person's mind, body, and spirit by outlining seven steps to a healthy life.

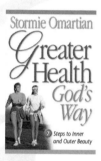

DITCH THE DIET AND THE BUDGET...
AND FIND A BETTER WAY TO LIVE
Cynthia Yates

Who wouldn't like a little more money and a little less weight? With her trademark warmth, humor, and common sense, award-winning humor columnist Cynthia Yates points readers to a better way to live.

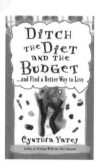

HARVEST HOUSE
PUBLISHERS